Clonidine workshop
Titisee 13–15 October 1983

Mild hypertension

Current controversies and new approaches

Edited by M. A. Weber and C. J. Mathias

With an introduction
by W. S. Peart

Contributions from

F. Alhenc-Gelas, L. Ceremużyński,
J. G. Collier, J. I. M. Drayer, S. S. Franklin,
G. P. Guthrie, Jr., K. Hayduk, K. Heilmann,
G. Mancia, C. J. Mathias, F. G. McMahon,
W. S. Peart, R. J. Polinsky, M. Rowland,
M. P. Sambhi, J. E. Shaw, M. Tuck,
M. A. Weber

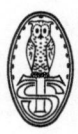 Steinkopff Verlag Darmstadt

Prof. M. A. Weber
Hypertension Center
Veterans Administration Center
5901 East 7th Street
Long Beach, California 90822
U.S.A.

Dr. C. J. Mathias M. B., B. S., D. Phil., M. R. C. P.
Senior Wellcome Fellow in Clinical Science,
Honorary Consultant Physician and
Senior Lecturer in Medicine, Medical Unit
St. Mary's Hospital Medical School
Norfolk Place, London W2 1PG
Great Britain

CIP-Kurztitelaufnahme der Deutschen Bibliothek

Mild hypertension : current controversies and new
approaches / [Clonidine Workshop, Titisee, 13 – 15
October 1983]. Ed. by M. A. Weber and C. J. Mathias.
With an introd. by W. S. Peart. Contributions from
F. Alhenc-Gelas . . . – Darmstadt : Steinkopff, 1984. –

ISBN 978-3-7985-0647-3   ISBN 978-3-642-87506-9 (eBook)
DOI 10.1007/978-3-642-87506-9

NE: Clonidine Workshop ‹1983, Oktober, Titisee›; Weber, Michael A. [Hrsg.]; Alhenc-Gelas, F. [Mitverf.]

Copyright © 1984 by Dr. Dietrich Steinkopff Verlag, GmbH & Co. KG, Darmstadt
Editorial Assistance: Juliane K. Weller − Production: Heinz J. Schäfer

Foreword

There is clear evidence that in severe hypertension lowering blood pressure, by drug therapy decreases the incidence of major cardiovascular events. Recent studies suggest that such benefit may also extend to patients with mild to moderate hypertension. The putative benefits of drugs may be offset, however, by their adverse effects and a prime example is the increased incidence of impotence and metabolic disorders in patients on thiazide diuretics. There is, therefore, a real need to look further into the therapy of patients with mild to moderate hypertension. The ideal drug in such patients would oppose the basic mechanisms responsible for the elevation in blood pressure, would prevent counter-regulatory responses and would have minimal side-effects in both the short-term and the long-term, the latter being of particular importance to younger patients.

These aspects were considered at the symposium "Mild hypertension. Current controversies and new approaches" held at Titisee in West Germany, October 13–15 in 1983.

The foundation for discussion was set with an exposition of the neural and hormonal regulation of blood pressure in normal man followed by a consideration of the possible pathophysiological mechanisms involved in patients with hypertension. Particular attention was focused on the central nervous system and on effects governed by activity of the peripheral nervous system as these may well provide further opportunities for logical therapeutic intervention in clinical hypertension. The current management of mild to moderate hypertension was then reviewed. Diuretics, β-adrenergic blockers, centrally acting anti-hypertensives, converting enzyme inhibitors and calcium antagonists were considered in relation to their use as either monotherapy or combination therapy. Attention was paid to the management of hypertension in patients with obesity, diabetes mellitus, ischaemic heart disease and the elderly, as in these groups, selective or modified therapeutic approaches may be necessary.

The final sessions of the symposium concentrated on novel strategies in therapy, as it was clear that in spite of the availability of potentially effective agents, there were undoubtedly limitations to their use. One approach is to use depot preparations of available drugs, the effects of which have already been well defined. Current research indicates that the transdermal route may offer some advantages in terms of ease of application, duration of action and maintenance of suitable plasma drug concentrations, particularly for agents whose actions are clearly related to drug concentrations. The first antihypertensive agent available in this form is clonidine, and recent trials with the transdermal form were presented and discussed. Early studies in patients with mild to moderate essential hypertension appear encouraging, but further work is needed both in relation to its effects on the skin and to the definition of its clinical niche in the management of hypertension.

The proceedings of this symposium represent a comprehensive view of the physiological and biochemical basis of blood pressure control, the possible mechanisms contributing to essential hypertension, the advantages and disadvantages of currently available drug therapy and a consideration of newer therapeutic approaches. The symposium, we feel, helped weld together basis concepts with newer therapeutic ideas and we would like to thank Dr. R. K. Rondel for meticulously organizing it and facilitating the editorial work. We hope that these proceedings will be of as much interest and guidance to you as the symposium was to us.

Christopher J. Mathias
Medical Unit
St. Mary's Hospital Medical School,
Norfolk Place
London W2 1PG
Great Britain

Michael A. Weber
Hypertension Center
Veterans Administration Center
Long Beach, Calif. 90822 U.S.A.

Contents

Advances in treatment
Chairman: M. P. Sambhi

Introduction:
Some neurological aspects of blood pressure control

W. S. Peart

It may at first seem strange that in a meeting on mild hypertension many of the papers should concern the nervous system. Such an emphasis arises naturally, however, from the recent resurgence of interest in the neurological control of the circulation. This introductory paper aims to pin-point some of the important neurological considerations and thus to form a framework for a more detailed discussion of the treatment of mild hypertension by subsequent contributors.

History

Our understanding of the role of the nervous system in cardiovascular control has developed over some 140 years (see review by Peart 1979). The term 'vasomotor nerves' was first used by Stelling in 1840 and their action on blood vessels was confirmed by the studies of Claude Bernard, Waller and Brown-Séquard in the 1850's. By the latter half of the 19th century growing knowledge of physiological chemistry and endocrinology had led to the ready acceptance of the concept that organs could release substances into the circulation. The demonstration by Oliver and Schafer of the pressor effects of an intravenous injection of an adrenal gland extract was of particular importance. Adrenaline was the first hormone to be purified (Abel and Crawford 1899), and subsequently to be synthesized (Stolz 1904; Dakin 1905). At this time Elliott first suggested that a sympathetic impulse might liberate adrenaline at the nerve ending, to act on the blood vessels. In 1907 Langley postulated the existence of a receptive area on muscle which would respond to the substance liberated from what we now know to be cholinergic nerve endings. Barger and Dale (1910) investigated the relationship between the Elliott hypothesis and the group of amines that they were then synthesizing and studying pharmacologically. In his retrospective assessment of their work, Dale (1965) remarked that he was too concerned with pointing out the differences between sympathetic action and the action of adrenaline to notice that noradrenaline fitted the requirements for the sympathetic neurotransmitter. It was not until Loewi (1921) demonstrated 'Acceleranstoff', released by stimulating the vasomotor nerves to the heart, that the chemical theory of neurotransmission received wide support. Although Cannon and Rosenblueth were still referring to the humoral effects of sympathetic nerve stimulation under the headings of sympathin E and I as late as 1933, by 1934 Bacq had suggested – on a critical assessment of previous work – that noradrenaline was likely to be the substance involved. In 1946 von Euler extracted noradrenaline from the splenic nerves. At that time, working in Gaddum's laboratory, I showed by parallel pharmacological assay that the substance that appeared in blood after sympathetic nerve stimulation was noradrenaline (Peart 1949).

1

The assessment of the activity of the sympathetic nervous system as opposed to its basic physiological mechanism, has followed two main lines. The first has attempted to correlate sympathetic nerve action with the appearance of noradrenaline in the blood stream and its metabolic products in the urine. The second has been an increasingly detailed study of sympathetic fibres and terminals. The latter approach has been the more rewarding. Since it has been applied centrally within the nervous system, as well as at the periphery, it has led to a much greater understanding of the mode of action of many different drugs. We know much more about the intimate workings of the synapse, however, than we do about the overall function of the sympathetic nervous system. Von Euler (1956) was one of the first to study patients with autonomic insufficiency. He and his colleagues showed two main abnormalities. A fluorescence method of catechol determination (von Euler and Floding 1956) showed these patients to have very low blood levels when either lying or standing. This was matched by very low levels of both free and conjugated forms of adrenaline and noradrenaline in the urine. At this time the full pattern of metabolic products in the urine was not known, but I remember using these observations in the diagnosis of patients with phaechromocytoma. The rat blood pressure preparation was used as the final assay of free amines. More recently, Mathias et al. (1975), working with patients with transected cervical cords, have demonstrated the failure of very low plasma noradrenaline levels to rise on tilting. These patients are, of course, without higher sympathetic outflow. Patients with phaeochromocytomas have a gross excess of catechols in the plasma. They may be differentiated from patients with other forms of hypertension by plasma assay. This has become a standard investigation in phaeochromocytoma along with assessment of the marked increase of metanephrines in the urine (Manger and Gifford 1977). Plasma catechol levels must be regarded as a very crude guide to the level of sympathetic nervous activity because of various factors which have emerged in relation to the release and subsequent fate of noradrenaline. This is particularly the case at the intermediate levels of sympathetic activity which are most interesting with respect to the control of the circulation.

Sympathetic pharmacology

Figure 1. is a diagram showing our present understanding of sympathetic pharmacology at both peripheral and central levels (see Stjärne et al. 1981 for background references). All the factors which affect the release of noradrenaline into the synaptic cleft may be classified as either stimulators or inhibitors. The major final event whereby a vesicle containing noradrenaline and other substances attaches itself to the membrane and liberates its contents by exocytosis, has been shown to depend upon the centry of calcium ions into the nerve ending. Once in the cleft, noradrenaline may follow a number of courses.
• It may attach to the $alpha_1$-receptor on the effector cell.
• It may re-enter the nerve ending (uptake 1), there to be metabolized by monoamine oxidase (MAO) to 3:4 dihydroxymandelic acid and subsequently to VMA (vanilyl mandelic acid); this re-uptake can be blocked by cocaine.
• It may diffuse in the cleft to stimulate $alpha_2$-prejunctional receptors which inhibit the release of noradrenaline.

2

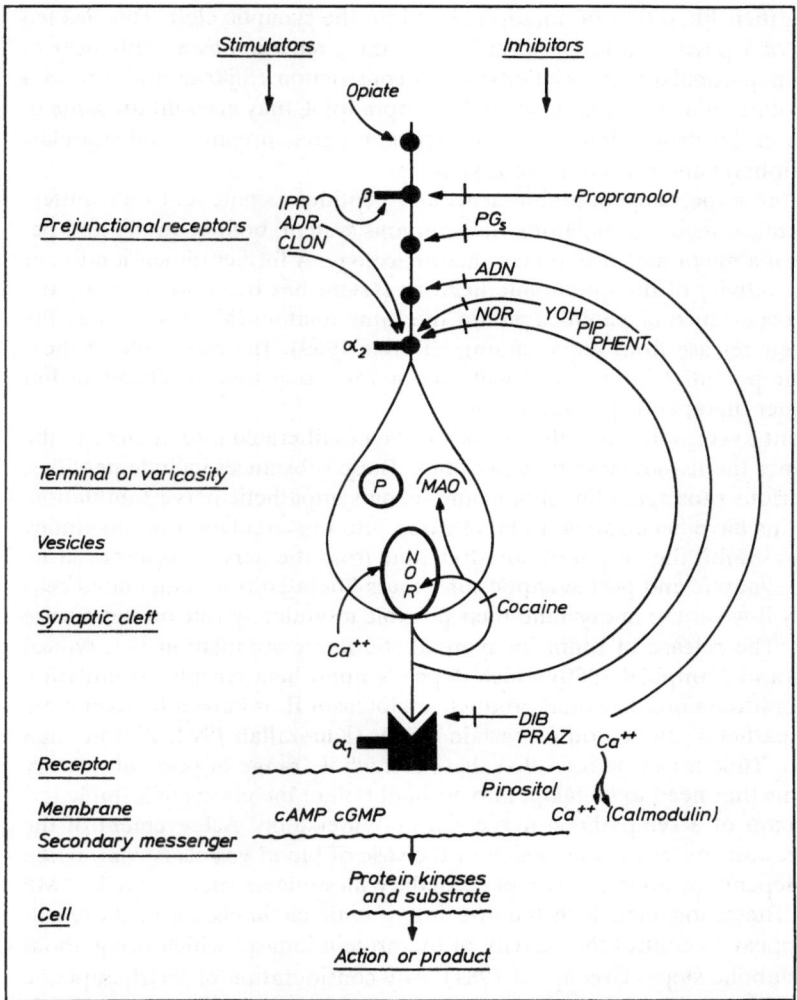

Fig. 1. Diagrammatic representation of α sympathetic nerve terminal, varicosity or equivalent structure in the brain.

Glossary: OPIATE (morphine or naloxone sensitive), IPR (isoprenaline), ADR (adrenaline), CLON (clonidine), P (neuropeptide) NOR (noradrenaline), MAO (monoamine oxidase), PGs (prostaglandins), ADN (adenosine), YOH (yohimbine), PIP (piperoxane), PHENT (phentolamine), DIB (dibenziline), PRAZ (prazosin), P. inositol (phosphatidyl inositol)

- Some may lodge on acceptor surfaces (uptake 2).
- The remainder enters the blood stream as an overflow, where it has distant effects, before it is converted to normetanephrine by catechol-*o*-methyl transferase (COMT).

Stimulation of the alpha$_1$-receptor may be blocked by dibenzyline, prazosin, or phentolamine, and of the alpha$_2$-receptor by yohimbine, piperoxane or phentolamine. The beta-prejunctional-receptors have been shown to respond to isoprenaline and adrenaline by increasing their liberation of noradrenaline into the synaptic cleft. This has led to the suggestion of a possible role for adrenaline in the circulation as an enhancer of sympathetic action particularly in relation to vasoconstriction (Stjärne and Brundin 1975). These receptors, which may be blocked by propranolol, may account for some of the cardiac action of this drug. Clonidine is an excellent alpha$_2$-prejunctional-stimulator in both the peripheral and central nervous systems.

The discovery of the importance of amino acids and peptides as potential transmitters or controllers of transmission in the autonomic nervous system, both centrally and peripherally, has been a major advance in neuropharmacology. A further dimension to our knowledge of the activity of the autonomic nervous system has been provided by the discovery of the occurrence of peptides within the same anatomical structures as the amines and of their release from nerve endings (Pearse 1969). The exact role of these peptides and their potential interactions will take a very long time to elucidate but there may be further therapeutic possibilities here.

It is most important to consider the influence of substances liberated into or close to the synaptic cleft or into the tissues close to varicosities. These substances include peptides, adenosine and various prostaglandins. For example, on sympathetic nerve stimulation, some prostaglandins have been shown to be released into the circulation of the kidney and secondarily to inhibit the output of noradrenaline from the nerve endings (Stjärne et al. 1981) These synaptic and post-synaptic substances liberated from innervated cells need careful study if we are to understand their possible modulating role on the release of noradrenaline. The release of renin by sympathetic nerve stimulation is a typical example (Keeton and Campbell 1980) which depends upon beta-receptor stimulation by the released noradrenaline. The final product, angiotensin II, is known to accentuate the effects of sympathetic stimulation on certain tissues (Khairallah 1972; Zimmerman and Gisslen 1968). Thus it can be seen that there is a whole range of post stimulatory modulating systems that need to be taken into account before the effects of a single impulse down the axon of a sympathetic nerve can be understood. Achievement of the end point of neurotransmitter release, which in the case of blood vessels is contraction or relaxation, is dependant upon a series of secondary messengers such as cyclic AMP and cyclic GMP. These, together, with the opening of ionic channels, particularly calcium channels, appear to control the activity of the protein kinases which bring about the important metabolic steps (Greengard 1981). Any consideration of the therapeutic effects of drugs on blood pressure must take into account their actions on the synapses and varicosities of the nervous system This is true even of the so-called calcium flux antagonists, notwithstanding the belief that calcium entry into the relevant smooth muscles may be of greater importance.

I shall now mention briefly some major aspects of the control of the circulation in man, each of which really deserves its own more detailed consideration.

Baroreceptor control

It is obvious that hypertension could not exist if the baroreceptors were effective in reducing high blood pressure over a prolonged period. I have argued (Peart 1980) that the experimental observations, in animals and in man, which show rapid adaptation of carotid sinus receptors to a high pressure (McCubbin et al. 1956), indicate that high pressure is not, by itself, a major controlling factor in the circulation. I think that circulatory adjustments are aimed at maintaining tissue flow above a certain minimum level, particularly to important areas like the brain and kidneys, and that baroreceptor mechanisms are especially important for raising the blood pressure from a low level and for modulating rapid changes. It is therefore more profitable to think of the circulation as maintaining tissue flow than as maintaining any particular level of pressure. Maintenance of pressure may be considered as a secondary phenomenon. The autoregulation of the circulation in response to raised blood pressure has been more difficult to demonstrate than that in response to lowered blood pressure, even though there is an experimental basis for expecting vasoconstriction in response to a raised blood pressure, as well as the perhaps more important vasodilation at low pressure. This, of course, is inherent in the original Bayliss concept (Bayliss 1902). To date, there have been very few therapeutic approaches to modification of the baroreceptor mechanisms, even though there have been many studies on the pharmacological responses of the carotid sinus reflex (Jones and Sleight 1981).

Humoral effects on the central nervous system

Until recently, the influence of the central nervous system on the circulation has been investigated largely by extirpation, blocking or stimulation of various areas, either anatomically or pharmacologically. It has become apparent that some effects on the blood pressure which were previously thought to be purely humoral in origin may be modified by the action of the central nervous system. This is perhaps most clearly shown in the case of phaeochromocytoma, where I certainly believed that most of the pressor effect was due to circulating noradrenaline, even though in the past it had frequently been pointed out that there was a discrepancy between the levels measured and the height of the blood pressure achieved. Maintenance of the blood pressure at a higher level by central nervous involvement undoubtedly occurs in many patients with phaeochromocytoma. This is suggested by the frequent failure of drugs such as phentolamine to reduce the pressure in such patients (Manger and Gifford 1977) and the fact that clonidine will do so (Bravo 1983). A central nervous component in the case of renal hypertension has also been suggested by similar responses to clonidine (Mathias et al. 1983). The comparison of central nervous and peripheral vascular actions adds another dimension to the interpretation of the action of direct competitive angiotensin blockers like saralasin, or indirect ones like captopril.

Mild hypertension

From a clinical point of view, hypertension is defined as that level of blood pressure which is likely to cause excess morbidity or mortality in the patient or the population being examined, within the next 5–10 years. In the case of mild hypertension, this usually means diastolic blood pressure between 90 and 105 mm Hg. Large scale trials of treatment are directed at patients whose blood pressures are within this range. The clinical problem (Peart 1981) concerns the advice one should give to the individual patient. Is it possible to give a risk factor to that individual, since all trials are based on large numbers and the overall results of the application of treatment? Is it possible to single out individuals who are at special risk unless they already show end organ damage? Blood pressure is the result of many forces, and considerable variability within an individual probably reflects the differing moment to moment activities of these different controlling factors. It is therefore not surprising that a competitive angiotensin II blocker, such as saralasin, may not lower the blood pressure of a normal individual on a diet containing 150 mmols of sodium daily, but will do so when the activity of the renin-angiotensin system is increased on a diet of 10 mmols of sodium daily. In this latter case a larger proportion of the prevailing pressure is due to the action of angiotensin.

Labile blood pressure and its implications cause a major problem to those who must decide on treatment of hypertension. I have always felt, therefore, that labile blood pressure is the description which should be applied and not that of labile or borderline hypertension, which is a diagnostic label with important implications for treatment (Peart 1980). Since 40% of the entrants to the Australian and MRC trials of treatment in 'mild hypertension' drop their blood pressure to the desired level on placebo treatment, this is a major consideration (Peart 1981). It is likely that the nervous system is a major contributory factor to the lability of blood pressure.

I hope that this introduction will provide a reasonable foundation for subsequent contributors. We are faced with the dilemma of therapeutic epidemiology versus clinical judgment. This is a subject of continuing controversy. Should whole populations of symptomless people (not patients) be treated with hypotensive drugs so as to reduce, in theory, the population risk; or should the individual be observed over time to assess his personal risk factors before the clinician makes a decision regarding treatment?

References

1 Abel JJ, Crawford AC (1899) Hoppe-Seyler's Z Physiol Chem 28:318.
2 Bacq ZM (1975) Chemical Transmission of Nerve Impulses. Pergamon Press, Oxford & New York
3 Barger G, Dale HH (1910) Chemical structure and sympathomimetic action of amines. J Physiol 41:19–59.
4 Bayliss WM (1902) On the local reactions of the arterial wall to changes of internal pressure. J Physiol 28:220–231.
5 Bernard C (1851) C R Soc Biol Les Fil 3:163.
6 Bravo EL (1983) Effects of clonidine on sympathetic function. Chest 83 (Suppl 2):369s–371s.
7 Brown-Séquard CE (1854) C R Acad Sci 38:72.
8 Cannon WB, Rosenblueth A (1933) Am J Physiol 104:557.
9 Dakin HD (1905) Proc R Soc London Ser B 76:491.
10 Dale HH (1965) Adventures in Physiology with excursions into autopharmacology: a selection from the scientific publications of Sir Henry Hallett Dale. The Wellcome Trust, London.
11 Elliott TR (1904) On the action of adrenalin. J Physiol (Lond) 31:20–21 p.
12 Euler US von (1946) Noradrenaline. CC Thomas, Springfield, Illinois.
13 Euler US von, Floding I (1956) Diagnosis of pheochromocytoma by fluorimetric estimation of adrenaline and noradrenaline in urine. Scand J Clin Lab Invest 8:288–295.
14 Greengard P (1981) Intracellular signals in the brain. The Harvey Lectures, 1980 75:277–331.
15 Jones JV, Sleight P (1981) Reflex control of the circulation in hypertensive humans. In: Abboud FM, Fozzard HA, Gilmore JP, Reis DJ (eds) Disturbances in Neurogenic Control of the Circulation. American Physiological Society, Bethesda, 161–175
16 Keeton TK, Campbell WB (1980) The pharmacologic alteration of renin release. Pharmacol Rev 32:81–227.
17 Khairallah PA (1972) Action of angiotensin on adrenergic nerve endings: inhibition of norepinephrine uptake. Fed Proc 31:1351–1357.

18 Langley JN (1907) J Physiol (Lond) 36:347
19 Loewi O (1921) Pflueger's Arch 189:239.
20 McCubbin JW, Green JH, Page IH (1956) Baroreceptor function in chronic renal hypertension. Circ Res 4:205–210.
21 Manger WM, Gifford RW Jr (1977) Pheochromocytoma. Springer Verlag, New York.
22 Mathias CJ, Christensen NJ, Corbett JL, Frankel HL, Goodwin TJ, Peart WS (1975) Plasma catecholamines, plasma renin activity and plasma aldosterone in tetraplegic man, horizontal and tilted. Clin Sci Molec Med 49:291–299.
23 Mathias CJ, Wilkinson A, Lewis PS, Peart WS, Sever PS, Snell ME (1983) Clonidine lowers blood pressure independently of renin suppression in patients with unilateral renal artery stenosis. Chest 83 (Suppl 2):357s–359s.
24 Oliver G, Schäfer EA (1894) J Physiol (Lond) 16:1 p.
25 Pearse AGE (1969) The cytochemistry and ultrastructure of polypeptide hormone-producing cells of the apud series and the embryologic, physiologic and pathologic implications of the concept. J Histochem Cytochem 17:303–313.
26 Peart WS (1949) The nature of splenic sympathin. J Physiol 108:491–501.
27 Peart WS (1979) Humors and hormones. The Harvey Lectures 1978 73:259–290.
28 Peart WS (1980) Concepts in hypertension. JR Coll Physicians Lond 14:141–152.
29 Peart WS (1981) The problem of treatment in mild hypertension. Clin Sci 61:402s–411s.
30 Stelling C (1867) Experimentelle Untersuchungen über den Einfluss des Nervus Depressor auf die Herzthätigkeit und den Blutdruck. Laakmann, Dorpat.
31 Stjärne L, Brundin J (1975) Dual adrenoceptor-mediated control of noradrenaline secretion from human vasoconstrictor nerves: facilitation by β-receptors and inhibition by α-receptors. Acta Physiol Scand 94:139–141.
32 Stjärne L, Hedqvist P, Lagercrantz H, Wennmalm A (eds) (1981) Chemical Neurotransmission, 75 years. Academic Press, London.
33 Stolz F (1904) Ber Dtsch Chem Ges 37:4149.
34 Waller AV (1853) C R Acad Sci 36:378.
35 Zimmerman BG, Gisslen J (1968) Pattern of renal vasoconstriction and transmitter release during sympathetic stimulation in presence of angiotensin and cocaine. J Pharmacol Exp Ther 163:320–329.

Correspondence:
W. S. Peart, MD, FRCP, FRS
Professor of Medicine
St. Mary's Hospital
London W2 1NY
U.K.

Central and peripheral control of blood pressure

Chairman: M. A. Weber

Central nervous system control of blood pressure

R. J. Polinsky

Introduction

Increased awareness of the effects on the central nervous system (CNS) of untreated hypertension has fostered a successful era of preventive medicine within neurology. The decline in mortality from stroke within the last decade is partly a result of early detection and treatment of hypertension. Conversely, the role of the CNS as a cause of hypertension is currently the focus of major research efforts in neuropharmacology. New classes and generations of antihypertensive drugs have been designed as a result of an increased understanding of the involvement of CNS in blood pressure control. One example is clonidine which, although initially developed as a nasal decongestant, has been successfully used as an antihypertensive and a pharmacological research tool. This paper will briefly review the role of the CNS in blood pressure control and the assessment of sympathetic neuronal function in man.

Autonomic neural organization

The parts of the nervous system responsible for blood pressure control are located in the more primitive, caudal areas of the brain. They control the physiological and hormonal mechanisms which contribute to overall regulation of blood pressure. It is primarily the baroreceptor reflex arc which makes acute adjustments of blood pressure and maintains circulatory homoeostasis. It responds rapidly and operates efficiently over a wide range of pressures. The autonomic nervous system is, in effect, a closed-loop feedback control system (Fig. 1); there are reflex pathways consisting of a sensor, central integration system and effector.

The afferent system

The location of the major baroreceptors in the carotid sinus and aortic arch allows the arterial pressure to the brain to be monitored (Spickler et al. 1967). These sensory receptors respond to pressure; increased pressure in the carotid sinus or aortic arch causes an increased firing frequency in the baroreceptor nerves. This increased activity can be maintained for prolonged periods if the pressure remains high (Diamond 1955). Afferent nerve fibres transmit this information to the brainstem central integration centres where an efferent response is generated to adjust vascular tone or cardiac function. In addition to the baroreceptors, there are several other types of peripheral sensors. Low-pressure cardiac mechanoreceptors sense atrial filling and thus provide an indication of the status of venous return to the heart (Paintal 1963). Chemoreceptors respond to changes in arterial oxygen (Eyzaguirre and Lewin 1961), carbon dioxide and

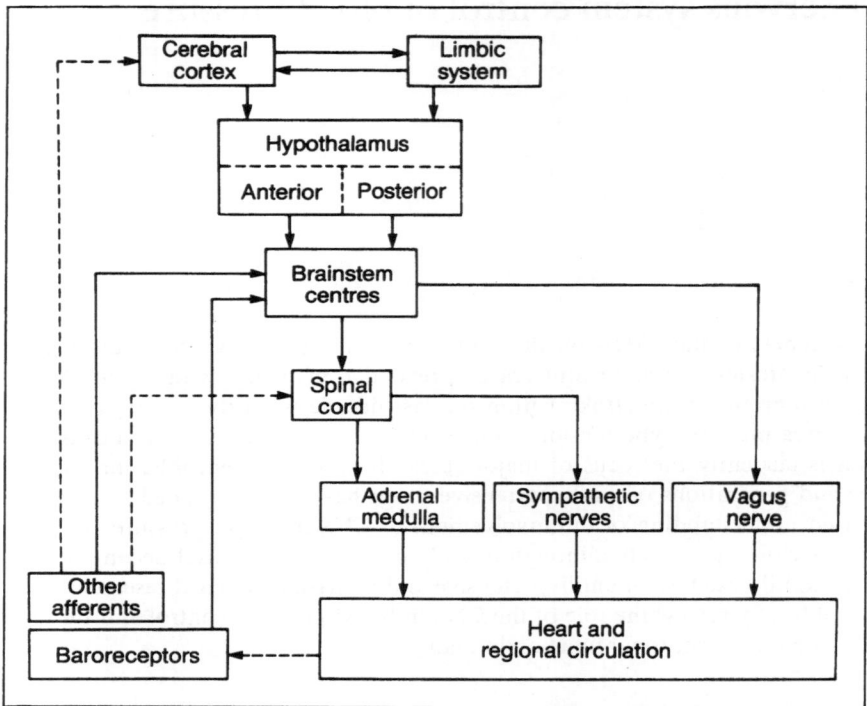

Fig. 1. Schematic diagram of central nervous system blood pressure control

pH (Hornbein et al. 1961). The phasic responses of pulmonary stretch receptors during respiration cause sinus arrhythmia.

CNS pathways

The nucleus of the tractus solitarius (NTS) in the medulla oblongata (Fig. 2) is the site of the first synapse of the afferent baroreceptor fibres which form part of the 9th and 10th cranial nerves (Humphrey 1967; Muira and Reis 1969). Although afferent input is widely dispersed through many polysynaptic pathways to numerous central integrative areas, the NTS projects directly to the spinal cord, parabrachial nucleus, nucleus ambiguus and hypothalamus (Loewy and Burton 1978; Loewy and McKellar 1980; Dampney 1981). Although recent findings dispute the existence of a discrete vasomotor center (VMC), this concept is, for simplicity, still used in discussion. The VMC receives inhibitory input from the NTS in contrast to the excitatory fibres which innervate the dorsal motor nucleus of the vagus (DMN) (Palkovits and Zaborszky 1977). Thus, increased activity of the baroreceptor afferents due to elevated blood pressure leads to diminished activity in the sympathetic efferent system and increased vagal tone. Higher centres involved in cardiovascular regulation include areas of the hypothalamus, basal ganglia, limbic system, and cerebral cortex (Korner 1971). Stimulation of the posterior hypothalamus leads to elevation of blood pressure (Przuntek et al. 1971) which is prob-

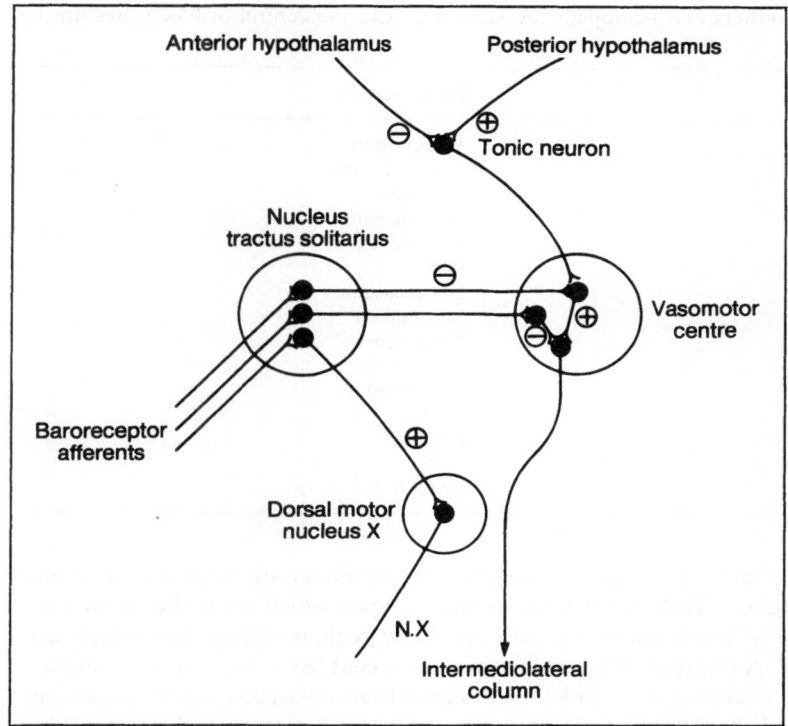

Fig. 2. Central nervous system pathways involved in cardiovascular control

ably mediated through an increase in the tonic activity of the VMC. The results of anterior hypothalamic stimulation are directly opposed to those of the posterior area (Hilton and Spyer 1971).

The efferent system

Efferent autonomic cardiovascular innervation is derived from large motor neuron pools in the DMN and the intermediolateral column of the spinal cord (ILC). Each of these neuronal groups receives input converging from many brain regions. ILC neurons are directly innervated by fibres from the NTS, ventrolateral reticular and ventral raphe nuclei, noradrenergic pontine neurons (Dampney 1981), and the hypothalamus (Blessing and Chalmers 1979). Pre-ganglionic sympathetic and vagal nerve fibres arise from the ILC and DMN, respectively, and together constitute the autonomic outflow to the peripheral ganglia.

Neuropharmacological considerations

The occurrence of different concentrations of putative neurotransmitters, together with their metabolites and synthetic and degradative enzymes, among specific brain nuclei

13

Table 1. Neurotransmitters and neuropeptides associated with the control of blood pressure by the CNS

Neurotransmitters	Neuropeptides
Noradrenaline	Vasopressin
Adrenaline	Neurophysins
Dopamine	Oxytocin
5-HT	Angiotensins
Histamine	Bradykinin
Acetylcholine	TRH
	Somatostatin
	Substance P
	Neurotensin
	Enkephalins
	β-Endorphin
	ACTH
	α-MSH
	VIP
	Gastrin

supports the notion that the levels of these neurotransmitters are related to neuronal activity in these regions. Techniques have been developed which allow the application of minute amounts of these substances into tiny brain regions so that their effects can be studied directly. A number of animal studies have enabled some neurotransmitters and neuropeptides (Table 1) to be linked with central cardiovascular control, and have either demonstrated their presence in the appropriate CNS regions and/or shown an effect on blood pressure when the substance is administered into the CNS (Palkovits 1981). Only the noradrenergic and serotonergic systems will be considered in this review.

Neurotransmitter systems

The cell bodies of noradrenergic neurons are mainly located in the pons and medulla (Loewy and McKellar 1980). There are both ascending and descending noradrenergic pathways. Noradrenergic neurons in the ventrolateral medulla, NTS and locus coeruleus play a key role in central blood pressure control. The main origin of the descending noradrenergic reticulospinal pathway is the locus coeruleus (Loewy and McKellar 1980; Dampney 1981). Although CNS administration of noradrenaline (NA) or stimulation of noradrenergic nuclei have generally caused depressor responses (Day and Roach 1974; Coote and MacLeod 1974), there are studies which demonstrate that noradrenergic neurons have an excitatory influence (Chalmers and Reid 1972; Doba and Reis 1973; Neumayr et al. 1974). This may be the input that tonically increases blood pressure. The functions of noradrenergic neurons may vary according to their location within the CNS.

Serotonergic neurons are grouped among the raphe nuclei of the medulla and pons, in the dorsal pons, and in the midbrain (Kuhn et al. 1980). Analogous to the noradrenergic system, there are also ascending and descending projections. The responses of the various serotonergic nuclei are not uniform.

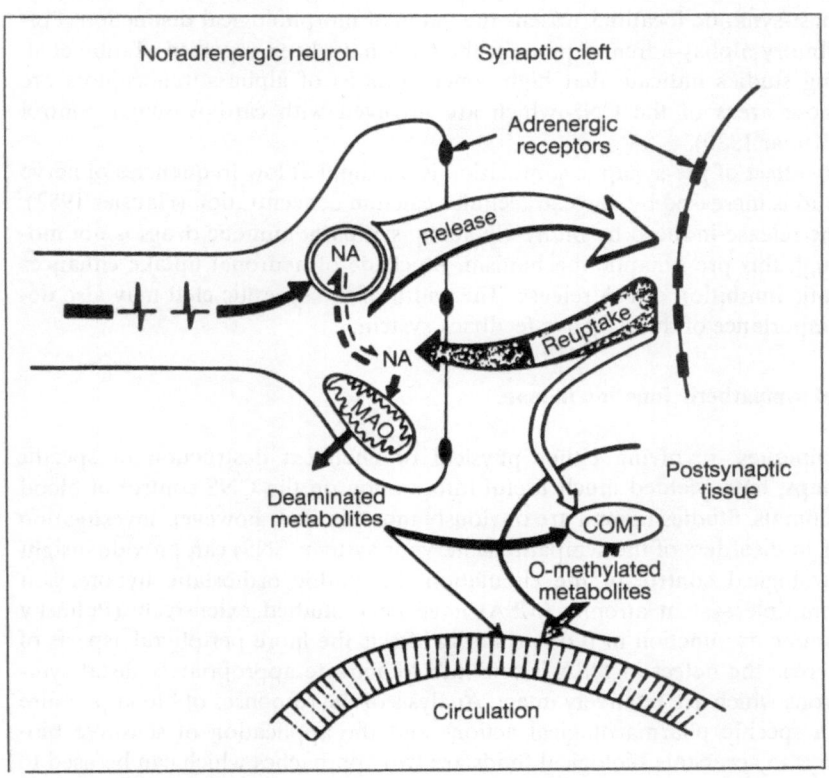

Noradrenergic neuron   Synaptic cleft

Adrenergic
receptors

Release

NA

Reuptake

NA

MAO

Postsynaptic
tissue

Deaminated
metabolites

COMT

O-methylated
metabolites

Circulation

lation is to inhibit further NA release (Langer et al. 1981). Neuronal uptake of NA into the cytoplasmic pool is the primary mode of terminating the action of endogenously released NA (Kopin 1972). A small amount of synaptic NA escapes into the plasma; some of this is metabolized to normetanephrine (NMN). Intraneuronal cytoplasmic NA is deaminated and subsequently metabolized to vanillylmandelic acid (VMA) and 3-methoxy, 4-hydroxyphenylglycol (MHPG). These characteristics of the noradrenergic neuron serve as a basis for developing biochemical and pharmacological indices of sympathetic function and also help to explain the mechanism of action of drugs which alter adrenergic function.

Adrenergic receptors

A number of distinct receptors, including two types of alpha-adrenoceptors, are associated with noradrenergic neurons. The morphological classification of peripheral adrenergic receptors is conceptually simple: pre-synaptic receptors inhibit NA release and post-synaptic receptors cause vasoconstriction (Langer 1977). An alternative schema is based on pharmacological differentiation: those receptors at which phenylephrine is more potent than clonidine are designated as alpha$_1$ in contrast to the alpha$_2$-receptors where the order of potency is reversed (Wikberg 1978). Although most of the receptors which inhibit NA release are of the alpha$_2$ type, the finding of both receptor subtypes at pre- and post-synaptic locations lessens the value of morphological distinction. Pre-synaptic inhibitory alpha$_2$-adrenoceptors in the CNS have been reported (Taube et al. 1977). Binding studies indicate that high concentrations of alpha-adrenoceptors are present in those areas of the CNS which are involved with cardiovascular control (Young and Kuhar 1980).

The inhibitory effect of pre-synaptic stimulation is maximal at low frequencies of nerve stimulation and is increased by low extracellular calcium concentration (Hausler 1982). Noradrenaline release induced by indirectly acting sympathomimetic drugs is not modulated through this pre-synaptic mechanism. Blockade of neuronal uptake enhances the pre-synaptic inhibition of NA release. The width of the synaptic cleft may also determine the importance of this negative feedback system.

Assessment of sympathetic function in man

Ablative techniques, involving either physical or chemical destruction of specific neuronal groups, have yielded much useful information on the CNS control of blood pressure in animals. Studies in man are obviously more limited; however, investigation of the deficits in disorders of the sympathetic nervous system (SNS) can provide insight into the neurological control of the circulation. Idiopathic orthostatic hypotension (IOH) and multiple system atrophy (MSA) have been studied extensively (Polinsky 1983). Autonomic dysfunction in IOH primarily affects the more peripheral aspects of the SNS, whereas the defect in MSA is a failure to activate appropriately distal sympathetic neurons which are relatively intact. Analysis of the responses of blood pressure to drugs with specific pharmacological actions and the application of sensitive biochemical assays to accessible biological fluids are two approaches which can be used to investigate SNS control of blood pressure in man.

Biochemical indices of SNS activity

Plasma NA levels correlate with sympathetic nerve activity (Wallin et al. 1981) and can be used to differentiate central and peripheral sympathetic dysfunction (Ziegler et al. 1977; Polinsky 1983). Low plasma NA levels in IOH result from post-ganglionic sympathetic neuronal dysfunction. Patients with MSA have normal supine plasma NA levels which do not increase adequately on standing, since post-ganglionic sympathetic neurons are not activated in response to postural stimuli. An increase in plasma NA has been reported in hypertensive patients (Engelman et al. 1970; Distler and Philipp 1980) but there are doubts about the validity and significance of this finding. It appears that a minority of hypertensive patients have delayed NA clearance (Esler et al. 1981); the elevation of plasma NA observed in the remaining patients is presumably the result of increased SNS activity.

The apportionment of urinary NA metabolites can be used to assess the integrity of peripheral noradrenergic neurons (Kopin et al. 1983). All metabolites are decreased in IOH since there are fewer remaining postganglionic sympathetic neurons. NMN is reduced out of proportion to VMA and MHPG in MSA; neuronal uptake and subsequent NA metabolism are normal but there is a decrease in the amount of NA released from the neurons, which leads to a reduction in the amount of NMN formed. Data for urinary NA metabolites in hypertensive patients have not been analyzed in this manner.

Measurement of urinary 6-hydroxymelatonin, a metabolite of melatonin, provides an index of pineal function, which is under the control of the beta-sympathetic nervous system (Tetsuo et al. 1981). Patients with IOH secrete diminished amounts of melatonin but their diurnal secretion pattern is normal. In most MSA patients, this diurnal fluctuation is lost and increased excretion of 6-hydroxymelatonin occurs during the day. This suggests that in MSA there is a CNS lesion which affects the control of pineal function.

Pressor responses

Exaggerated increases of blood pressure are observed in both IOH and MSA patients in response to intravenous NA and angiotensin, as illustrated in Fig. 4 (Polinsky et al. 1981). However, only IOH patients manifest a shift-to-the-left of their NA dose-response curves, which indicates true adrenergic receptor supersensitivity. The non-specific increase in slope is due to defective baroreceptor modulation of blood pressure. These findings are similar to the differences in sensitivity to sympathomimetic amines which are observed in animals after denervation and decentralization (Trendelenberg 1963). Decentralization does not alter the response to indirectly acting sympathomimetic drugs. Denervation causes an increase in receptor sensitivity to NA, accompanied by a loss of the response to indirectly acting sympathomimetics. The increment in plasma NA following intravenous tyramine is significantly reduced in IOH; it is not completely abolished because the lesion is incomplete. An exaggerated increase in blood pressure with NA has been reported in hypertensive patients (Distler and Philipp 1980); the mechanism of this response is unclear.

The response of blood pressure to clonidine depends on the nature and location of the SNS dysfunction. Clonidine lowers blood pressure primarily through a central mechanism which involves stimulation of presynaptic receptors (Isaac 1980). This causes a re-

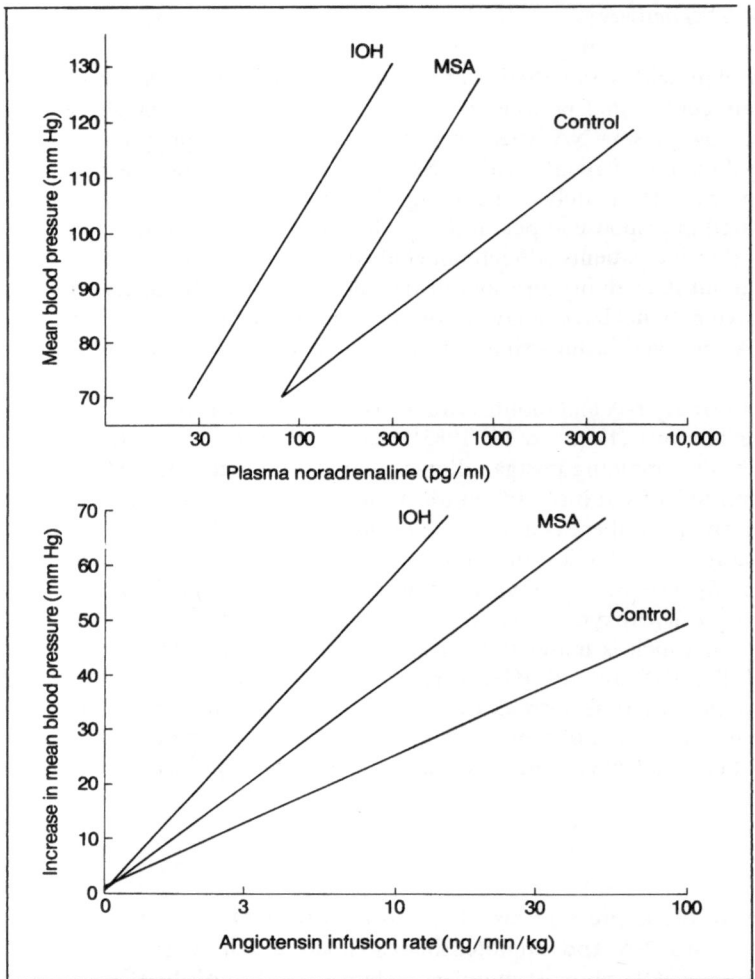

Fig. 4. Blood pressure responses to intravenous noradrenaline (upper) and angiotensin II (lower) in control subjects and patients with idiopathic orthostatic hypotension (IOH) and multiple system atrophy (MSA)

duction in sympathetic tone with a concomitant decrease in plasma NA levels. In IOH patients with efferent sympathetic dysfunction there may be no change in blood pressure following oral clonidine (Reid 1983). However, a pressor response has also been observed and utilized for the treatment of IOH (Robertson et al. 1983). This elevation of blood pressure may be due to peripheral vasoconstriction in the venous capacitance system. There is no blood pressure response to clonidine in tetraplegic patients (Mathias and Frankel 1983); in this situation the connection between the central integration system and postganglionic fibres has been severed. In contrast, afferent autonomic neuropathy does not alter the usual hypotensive response to clonidine (Reid 1983).

CSF studies

MHPG is the major metabolite of NA within the CNS. Recently, it has been shown that a proportion of MHPG in the CSF is derived from free plasma MHPG, which readily crosses the blood-brain barrier (Kopin et al. 1983). Levels of MHPG in the CSF can be used as an index of central NA metabolism if they are corrected for the contribution from plasma. Both IOH and MSA patients have low MHPG levels in the CSF but only IOH patients have diminished plasma-free MHPG (Polinsky et al. 1983). The corrected CSF MHPG level is only lower than normal in MSA patients, which indicates CNS noradrenergic dysfunction. Elevated CSF MHPG levels in hypertensive patients have been reported to be reduced by clonidine (Saran et al. 1978), but the CSF MHPG levels were not corrected. Levels of NA in the CSF are elevated in an least some patients with hypertension (Lake et al. 1981). However, the origin and disposition of NA in the CSF have not been clearly defined. The levels of other neurotransmitters and metabolites in the CSF have not been systematically investigated in these disorders.

Implications for synaptic pharmacotherapy

Modulation of the control of blood pressure by the CNS can be achieved through the development of drugs which pass easily across the blood-brain barrier and alter the outflow of the autonomic nervous system. The anatomical, biochemical, and pharmacological aspects of central blood pressure control discussed above provide a theoretical framework for understanding CNS mechanisms of drug action. Evaluation of the biochemical and pharmacological consequences of antihypertensive therapy may provide insight into the clinical limitations of these drugs. The blood pressure responses to specific drugs in patients with well-characterized lesions of the SNS can be used to confirm the site and mechanism of action of these drugs in man. Assessment of sympathetic function in other diseases may reveal additional applications for centrally acting drugs that modify adrenergic transmission. The importance of the noradrenergic system in central blood pressure control has been emphasized in this paper. Drugs may affect noradrenergic transmission by modifying neuronal and synaptic processes. Neuronal release and reuptake of NA as well as the spectrum of pre- and post-synaptic receptors, are potential targets for centrally acting drugs. For example, a reduction in sympathetic tone results from blockade of post-synaptic receptors or stimulation of pre-synaptic receptors. Although a decrease in neuronal reuptake increases the level of NA in the synaptic cleft, this increased NA inhibits further NA secretion by stimulating the inhibitory feedback control. It is only after the pre-synaptic receptors become subsensitized that neuronal uptake blockade effectively alters adrenergic transmission. This may explain the delay in clinical response which is observed to follow treatment with tricyclic antidepressants. The ability of a drug to block post-synaptic receptors and stimulate pre-synaptic receptors would be expected to enhance its potential to reduce sympathetic tone. The balance between alpha$_1$- and alpha$_2$-receptors varies within different tissues and probably within different brain regions. Hence, a drug that is more specific in its action might exhibit a more predictable response pattern.

The anatomical distribution of alpha-adrenoceptors in the hypothalamus, brainstem, and spinal cord provides multiple sites at which adrenergic activity can be altered. Unfortunately, the situation is complicated by the antagonistic responses which may be mediated by the same neurotransmitter in the hypothalamus. In addition, the brainstem contains several populations of noradrenergic neurons; some areas are involved with tonic blood pressure regulation while others participate in the baroreceptor reflex pathway. Other central sites of action may produce side-effects associated with the desired effects on blood pressure. Thus, it is important to determine the CNS distribution of a centrally acting drug.

A clearer definition of the involvement of the CNS in the genesis of hypertension would facilitate the design of more specific therapeutic approaches. An ideal centrally acting antihypertensive drug should:

- be highly soluble in lipids
- decrease sympathetic tone
- facilitate vagal activity
- not affect the reflex control of blood pressure
- have a limited distribution in the CNS
- be effective at low doses.

As an increased understanding of the role of other neurotransmitter and neuropeptide systems emerges, it may be possible to develop alternative strategies for controlling blood pressure through central mechanisms.

References

1 Blessing WW, Chalmers JP (1979) Direct projections of catecholamine (presumably dopamine-containing) neurons from hypothalamus to spinal cord. Neurosci Lett 11:35–40.
2 Chalmers JP, Reid JL (1972) Participation of central noradrenergic neurones in arterial baroreceptor reflexes in the rabbit. A study with intracisternally administered 6-hydroxydopamine. Circ Res 31:789–804.
3 Coote JH, MacLeod VH (1974) The influence of bulbospinal monoaminergic pathways on sympathetic nerve activity. J Physiol (Lond) 241:453–475.
4 Dahlstrom A, Fuxe K (1965) Evidence for the existence of monoamine neurons in the central nervous system. II. Experimentally induced changes in the intraneuronal amine levels of bulbospinal neuron systems. Acta Physiol Scand 64 (Suppl 274):1–36.
5 Dampney RAL (1981) Functional organization of central cardiovascular pathways. Clin Exp Pharmac Physiol 8:241–259.
6 Day MD, Roach AG (1974) Central α- and β-adrenoceptors modifying arterial blood pressure and heart rate in conscious cats. Br J Pharmac 51:325–333.
7 Diamond J (1955) Observations on the excitation by acetylcholine and by pressure of sensory receptors in the cat's carotid sinus. J Physiol 130:513–532.
8 Distler A, Philipp T (1980) Role of sympathetic nervous system in essential hypertension. Contrib Nephrol 23:150–157.
9 Doba N, Reis DJ (1973) Acute fulminating neurogenic hypertension produced by brainstem lesions in the rat. Circ Res 32:584–593.
10 Engelman K, Portnoy B, Sjoerdsma A (1970) Catecholamines – cyclic AMP-angiotension receptors. Plasma catecholamine concentrations in patients with hypertension. Circ Res 27 (Suppl 1):141–146.
11 Esler M, Jackman G, Bobik A, Leonard P, Kelleher D, Skews H, Jennings G, Korner P (1981) Norepinephrine kinetics in essential hypertension: Defective neuronal uptake of norepinephrine in some patients. Hypertension 3:149–156.
12 Eyzaguirre C, Lewin J (1961) Effect of different oxygen tensions on the carotid body in vitro. J Physiol 159:238–250.

13 Guyton AC, Hall JE, Lohmeier TE, Jackson TE, Kastner PR (1981) Blood pressure regulation: basic concepts. Fed Proc 40:2252–2256.
14 Häusler G (1982) Central α-adrenoceptors involved in cardiovascular regulation. J Cardiovasc Pharmacol 4:S72–S76.
15 Hilton SM, Spyer KM (1971) Participation of the anterior hypothalamus in the baroreceptor reflex. J Physiol 218:271–293.
16 Hornbein TF, Griffo ZJ, Roos A (1961) Quantitation of chemoreceptor activity: interrelation of hypoxia and hypercapnia. J Neurophysiol 24:561–568.
17 Humphrey DR (1967) Neuronal activity in the medulla oblongata of cat evoked by stimulation of the carotid sinus nerve. In: Kezdi P (ed.) Baroreceptors and Hypertension. Proceedings of International Symposium, Dayton, Ohio, 16–17 November 1965. Pergamon Press, Oxford, 131–168.
18 Isaac L (1980) Clonidine in the central nervous system: site and mechanism of hypotensive action. J Cardiovasc Pharmacol 2 (Suppl 1):S5–S19.
19 Kopin IJ (1972) Metabolic degradation of catecholamines. The relative importance of different pathways under physiological conditions and after administration of drugs. Handbook Exp Pharmacol 33:270–279.
20 Kopin IJ, Gordon EK, Jimerson DC, Polinsky RJ (1983) Relation between plasma and cerebrospinal fluid levels of 3-methoxy-4-hydroxyphenylglycol. Science 219:73–75.
21 Kopin IJ, Polinsky RJ, Oliver JA, Oddershede IR, Ebert MH (1983) Urinary catecholamine metabolites distinguish different types of sympathetic neuronal dysfunction in patients with orthostatic hypotension. J Clin Endocrinol Metab 57:632–637.
22 Korner PI (1971) Integrative neural cardiovascular control. Physiol Rev 51:312–367.
23 Kuhn DM, Wolf WA, Lovenberg W (1980) Review of the role of the central serotonergic neuronal system in blood pressure regulation. Hypertension 2:243–255.
24 Lake CR, Gullner HG, Polinsky RJ, Ebert MH, Ziegler MG, Bartter FC (1981) Essential hypertension: central and peripheral norepinephrine. Science 211:955–957.
25 Langer SZ (1977) Presynaptic receptors and their role in the regulation of transmitter release. Br J Pharmacol 60:481–497.
26 Langer SZ, Massingham R, Shepperson NB (1981) α_1- and α_2-receptor subtypes: relevance to antihypertensive therapy. In: Buckley JP, Ferrario CM (eds) Central Nervou System Mechanisms in Hypertension, Perspectives in Cardiovascular Research, Vol. 6, Raven Press, New York, 161–170.
27 Loewy AD, Burton H (1978) Nuclei of the solitary tract: efferent projections to the lower brain stem and spinal cord of the cat. J Comp Neurol 181:421–450.
28 Loewy AD, McKellar S (1980) The neuroanatomical basis of central cardiovascular control. Fed Proc 39:2495–2503.
29 Mathias CJ, Frankel HL (1983) Autonomic failure in tetraplegia. In: Bannister R (ed.) Autonomic failure. A textbook of clinical disorders of the autonomic nervous system. Oxford University Press, Oxford, 453–488.
30 Muira M, Reis DJ (1969) Termination and secondary projections of carotid sinus nerve in the cat brain stem. Am J Physiol 217:142–153.
31 Neumayr RJ, Hare BD, Franz DN (1974) Evidence for bulbospinal control of sympathetic preganglionic neurones by monoaminergic pathways. Life Sci 14:793–806.
32 Paintal AS (1963) Vagal afferent fibers. Ergeb Physiol Biol Chem Exp Pharmakol 52:74–156.
33 Palkovits M (1981) Neuropeptides and biogenic amines in central cardiovascular control mechanisms. In: Buckley JP, Ferrario CM (eds) Central Nervous System Mechanisms in Hypertension. Perspectives in Cardiovascular Research, Vol. 6, Raven Press, New York, 73–87.
34 Palkovits M, Zaborsky L (1977) Neuroanatomy of central cardiovascular control. Nucleus tractus solitarii: afferent and efferent neuronal connections in relation to the baroreceptor reflex arc. In: Dejong W, Provoost AP, Shapiro AP (eds) Progress in Brain Research, Vol 47, Hypertension and Brain Mechanisms. Elsevier, Amsterdam, 9–34.
35 Polinsky RJ (1983) Pharmacologic responses and biochemical changes in progressive autonomic failure. In: Bannister R (ed) Autonomic failure. A textbook of clinical disorders of the autonomic nervous system. Oxford University Press, Oxford, 201–236.
36 Polinsky RJ, Kopin IJ, Ebert MH, Weise V (1981) Pharmacologic distinction of different orthostatic hypotension syndromes. Neurology 31:1–7.

37 Polinsky RJ, Jimerson DC, Kopin IJ (1984) Chronic autonomic failure: CSF and plasma 3-methoxy-4-hydroxyphenylglycol. Neurology (in press).

38 Przuntek H, Guimaraes S, Philippu A (1971) Importance of adrenergic neurons of the brain for a rise of blood pressure evoked by hypothalamic stimulation. Naunyn Schmiedebergs Arch Pharmacol 271:311–319.

39 Reid JL (1983) Central and peripheral autonomic control mechanisms. In: Bannister R (ed.) Autonomic failure. A textbook of clinical disorders of the autonomic nervous system. Oxford University Press, Oxford, 17–35.

40 Robertson DL, Goldberg MR, Hollister AS, Wade D, Robertson RM (1983) Clonidine raises blood pressure in serve idiopathic orthostatic hypotension. Am J Med 74:193–200.

41 Saran RK, Sahuja RC, Gupta NN, Hasan M, Bhargava KP, Shanker K, Kishor K (1978) 3-methoxy-4-hydroxyphenylglycol in cerebrospinal fluid and vanillylmandelic acid in urine of humans with hypertension Science 200:317–318.

42 Spickler JW, Kezdi P, Geller E (1967) Transfer characteristics of the carotid sinus pressure control system. In: Kezdi P (ed) Baroreceptors and hypertension. Proceedings of International Symposium, Dayton, Ohio, 16–17 November 1965. Pergamon Press, Oxford, 31–40.

43 Taube HD, Starke K, Borowski E (1977) Presynaptic receptor systems on the noradrenergic neurones of rat brain. Naunyn Schmiedeberg's Arch Pharmacol 299:123–141.

44 Tetsuo M, Polinsky RJ, Markey SP, Kopin IJ (1981) Urinary 6-hydroxymelatonin excretion in patients with orthostatic hypotension. J Clin Endocrinol Metab 53:607–610.

45 Trendelenburg U (1963) Supersensitivity and subsensitivity to sympathomimetic amines. Pharmacol Rev 15:225–276.

46 Wallin BG, Sundlöf G, Eriksson B-M, Dominiak P, Grobecker H, Lindblad L-E (1981) Plasma noradrenaline correlates to sympathetic muscle nerve activity in normotensive man. Acta Physiol Scand 111:69–73.

47 Wikberg J (1978) Differentiation between pre- and postjunctional α-receptors in guinea pig ileum and rabbit aorta. Acta Physiol Scand 103:225–239.

48 Young WS, Kuhar MJ (1980) Noradrenergic α_1- and α_2-receptors: light microscopic autoradiographic localization. Proc Natl Acad Sci USA 77:1696–1700.

49 Ziegler MG, Lake CR, Kopin IJ (1977) The sympathetic-nervous-system defect in primary orthostatic hypotension. N Engl J Med 296:293–297.

Correspondence:
Ronald J. Polinsky, M.D.
N.I.N.C.D.S.
National Institutes of Health
Bethesda, Maryland 20205, USA

Discussion

WEBER:
Is clonidine used in patients with idiopathic orthostatic hypotension? Is there any therapeutic benefit and if so can you speculate on the mechanism?

POLINSKY:
We have not used clonidine. Other workers have used it and found a relationship between plasma noradrenaline levels (which reflect peripheral sympathetic activity) and those patients who are responders. In patients with some remaining central sympathetic tone there may be a fall in blood pressure since clonidine may block residual sympathetic activity. Clonidine however is a weak agonist postsynaptically in addition to being a presynaptic alpha$_2$-agonist. Alpha$_2$-receptors may also be present postsynaptically with different functions to presynaptic receptors. In patients without sympathetic activity, therefore, these peripheral effects of clonidine may result in a pressor response.

GUTHRIE:
From your dose-response pressor curves you state that your patients with autonomic insufficiency appear to have diminished baroreflex function. Have you assessed this directly?

POLINSKY:
No, but we have looked at results from the Valsalva manoeuvre, cold pressor test and other relatively crude assessments. We will be studying baroroflex function, however, using intra-arterial recordings with neck suction and other approaches.

COLLIER:
Is it correct that noradrenaline increases blood pressure if given in certain brain regions but lowers it in other places?

POLINSKY:
Some studies indicate that noradrenaline administered centrally produces depressor responses while other studies indicate pressor responses. The area looked at most carefully has been the hypothalamus: if instilled into the posterior hypothalamus there is a pressor response and in the anterior hypothalamus a depressor response, although both are mediated by an alpha-adrenergic receptor.

COLLIER:
Are there noradrenergic nerves there? Could this happen physiologically? Could there be nerves which release noradrenaline at the sites at which you give noradrenaline?

POLINSKY:
These are not our studies but I understand that the sites where noradrenaline was administered are in the same areas as those where noradrenergic pathways end.

MATHIAS:
Do you have any data on what happens to CSF and plasma MHPG levels when you give clonidine to either normal or hypertensive individuals?

POLINSKY:
We have not studied that. There was a study about 6 years ago from New York. They had observed elevated MHPG levels in the CSF of patients with hypertension which were lowered by clonidine. They did not, however, do the corrections for their levels as we do. It is possible that they were observing a depression of either peripheral or central MHPG. We need to go back and look at MHPG levels in the CSF of patients who have been given clonidine, using our principles of analysis, to see whether it is actually the central portion that goes down rather than the peripheral portion.

Blood pressure control and the peripheral sympathetic nervous system

C. J. Mathias

Introduction

The activity and final effects exerted by the peripheral sympathetic nervous system depend not only on central control mechanisms but also on a number of modulatory peripheral influences. I shall address myself to those peripheral effects which relate to cardiovascular function and in particular to blood pressure control. I shall outline the basic principles which govern such activity and provide examples, based mainly on clinical studies, which have provided a greater awareness of the functioning of this system in man.

The sympathetic nervous system

The sympathetic nervous system is essentially an efferent system. Pathways which traverse the cervical spinal cord descend from the brain. They synapse in the intermediolateral cell columns usually in the thoracic and upper lumbar segments of the spinal cord. From these cell masses arise myelinated preganglionic fibres which pass along the anterior nerve roots to the paravertebral sympathetic ganglia. Unmyelinated postganglionic fibres are distributed from these ganglia to the heart, arteries, veins and other effector organs. The adrenal gland, however, is an exception as it has mainly preganglionic fibres to the chromaffin cells. The sympathetic postganglionic fibres appear to be largely vasoconstrictor in nature and debate continues about the presence of sympathetic vasodilatatory pathways. Sympathetic activation usually causes an elevation in blood pressure, which implies an increase in peripheral vascular resistance and thus vasoconstriction in either the entire vascular tree or a major proportion of it. Certain stimuli, however, cause constriction in one bed and dilatation in another. Higher mental activity, for instance, which usually raises blood pressure, is consistently accompanied by dilatation in forearm vessels (Brod et al. 1959) but constriction in the dorsal veins of the hand (Fig. 1). The precise central control areas and the mechanisms which determine these responses in man are still not clearly defined. It is likely that in certain organs such differences relate to their specific physiological and perfusion needs.

Peripheral stimuli

The major peripheral sensors responsible for the fine control of blood pressure are the aortic, carotid and cardiopulmonary receptors. These are pressoreceptors or mechanoreceptors, although the actual activating stimulus is stretch and distension. A number of approaches have been used to study such receptors, including drugs (vasoconstrictors like phenylephrine and vasodilators like glyceryl trinitrate), neck suction

24

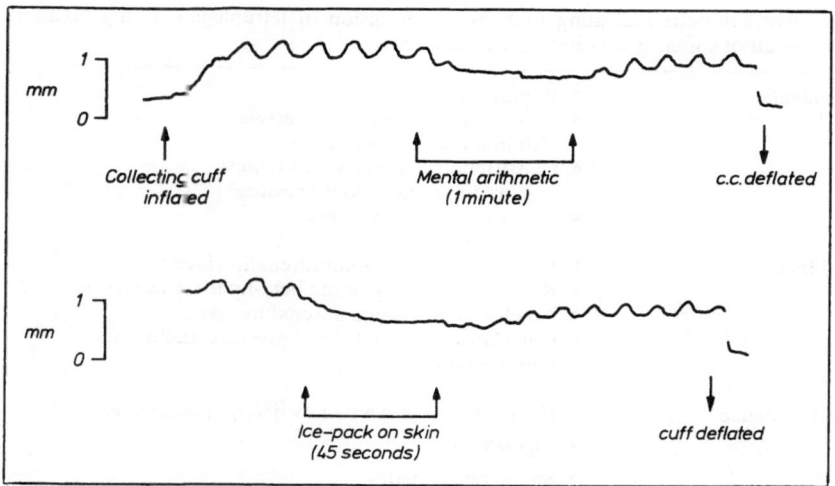

Fig. 1. Reduction in hand vein diameter during mental arithmetic and with an ice-pack on the skin, measured with a light-weight linear transducer. The technique enables rapid changes to be measured accurately (data from da Costa, Mathias and Peart)

(which stimulates carotid receptors) and lower body negative pressure (which mainly stimulates cardiopulmonary receptors). The final response exerted by such receptor stimulation depends not only on afferent impulses but also on intracerebral synaptic connections and on peripheral effector systems exerted by the parasympathetic system (to the heart) and the sympathetic system (to both heart and blood vessels). Abnormalities of these baroreflex pathways have been documented in hypertensive patients, but the precise sites of the lesions have not been demonstrated and it is not known whether they are the cause of or a consequence of hypertension.

A number of afferent stimuli from receptors in skin and muscle are relayed to the cerebral cortex and then influence brain stem cardiovascular centres. In man, activation of these receptors by low skin temperature or isometric exercise, rapidly elevates blood pressure. In tetraplegics with transected cervical cords, this rise in blood pressure does not occur if the stimulation has been initiated in innervated areas above the lesion. This indicates that both cerebral integration and descending bulbospinal pathways are necessary for the final responses. Cerebral activity, caused for instance by mental arithmetic, does not as a rule, raise blood pressure in tetraplegics (Corbett et al. 1971). There are exceptions, however, as tetraplegics trained by means of biofeedback techniques (Pickering et al. 1977) can raise their blood pressure by a conditioned, voluntary withdrawal of vagal tone which elevates heart rate. The rise in blood pressure appears to be secondary to an elevated cardiac output associated with a fixed peripheral vascular resistance. These effects are abolished by atropine, which further establishes the role of the vagus in this response. In normal subjects, mental stress, such as fear, may occasionally cause bradycardia and vasodilatation leading to circulatory collapse. Atropine may prevent the bradycardia but not the hypotension (Lewis 1932). In certain situations therefore, vasodilator pathways, involving neurotransmitters not yet determined, may be activated in preference to sympathetic vasoconstrictor pathways.

Table 1. Summary of evidence indicating that the hypertension in tetraplegics during bladder stimulation is the result of spinal sympathetic reflex activity

Physiological evidence	• Rapidity of onset • Constriction of resistance vessels (fall in forearm blood flow) • Constriction of capacitance vessels (rise in occluded venous pressure) • Increase in stroke volume
Biochemical evidence	• Elevation in plasma noradrenaline levels • Rise in plasma dopamine beta-hydroxylase levels • No change in plasma adrenaline levels • Correlation between blood pressure and plasma noradrenaline
Pharmacological evidence	Hypertension prevented by drugs at these sites.
Afferent	• Lignocaine
Spinal	• Spinal anaesthetics • Clonidine* and reserpine* • Phenol or alcohol
Ganglia	• Ganglion blockers
Sympathetic neuroeffector junction	• Guanethidine • Phenoxybenzamine

* may have actions at other sites

A number of visceral afferents are capable of inducing substantial circulatory effects at a spinal level and are unmasked in patients with absent cerebral sympathetic control. Patients with cervical or high thoracic cord transection readily elevate their blood pressure, at times to extremely high levels, during stimulation of the urinary bladder or other viscera. In them, reflex activity along the entire sympathetic chain, is triggered by a localized stimulus over a few dermatomes which causes widespread vasoconstriction and thus hypertension. Physiological, biochemical and pharmacological studies confirm that these effects are secondary to uninhibited spinal sympathetic reflex activity (Mathias and Frankel 1983, Table 1). In these patients the afferent and vagal efferent limbs of the sinoaortic baroreflex are intact, and are activated, as bradycardia often occurs. This, however, is not sufficient to prevent the rise in blood pressure. The role of the vagus though, is not entirely inconsequential, as blockade with atropine elevates blood pressure to an even greater level. To what extent visceral afferents influence blood pressure in normal and hypertensive man is not known.

Neurochemistry

The elucidation of the biochemistry and pharmacology of the peripheral sympathetic nervous system has considerably advanced our understanding of its function. Acetylcholine is the neurotransmitter at sympathetic ganglia and its influence over peripheral sympathetic nervous activity has been clearly demonstrated by the efficacy of ganglion blockers, the earliest drugs used in the management of severe hypertension. Numerous undesirable effects, however, have reduced clinical interest in such agents. Greater attention has been focused on the sympathetic neuroeffector junction. The key transmitter here is noradrenaline, whose release depends on a number of factors (Smith 1973). In resting normal subjects neuronal release partly depends on tonic impulses from brain stem centres which contribute to the neurogenic component of peripheral vascular resistance. This is absent in completely transected tetraplegics, who have a lower basal blood pressure and lower plasma noradrenaline levels than normal subjects (Mathias et al. 1976). Similar effects may be induced in normal subjects by the centrally acting sympatholytic agent clonidine (Wing et al. 1977), which in tetraplegics has no further effects in the basal state (Reid et al. 1977).

There are now sensitive and specific assays for measuring noradrenaline in plasma, which initially raised hopes of providing a reliable index of sympathetic nervous activity. Plasma noradrenaline levels are, however, the result of a large number of events occurring in and around the neuroeffector junction. When noradrenaline is released it acts upon alpha-1-adrenoceptors, but part of it is taken up by neuronal membrane uptake processes (uptake I) or extraneuronal processes (uptake II), while some is metabolized by enzymes such as monoamine oxidase (MAO) and catechol-o, methyltransferase (COMT); the remaining portion passes into the circulation. These are some of the factors which make it difficult to assess the putative role of the sympathetic nervous system in essential hypertension on the basis of plasma catecholamine levels alone. The neuronal release of noradrenaline is accompanied by a proportional release of dopamine-beta-hydroxylase (Weinshilboum et al. 1971). This enzyme is not subject to the inactivating and uptake processes of noradrenaline and it was originally thought to be a potentially ideal marker of sympathetic neuronal activity. This, however, has not been realized mainly because genetic factors markedly influence circulating levels. Other enzymes, such as MAO in platelets and COMT in erythrocytes, appear also to be genetically determined. Since many patients with essential hypertension have a strong familial basis the possibility remains that measurement of such enzymes may provide further information on the monoamine system in such patients and also on their ability to handle drugs which influence the system (Weinshilboum 1983).

Receptors

On the sympathetic nerve terminal are presynaptic receptors, one of which, the alpha-2-adrenoreceptor, can be activated by neuronally released noradrenaline. This appears to inhibit release of the neurotransmitter. To what extent this mechanism plays a physiological role in the modulation of peripheral sympathetic nervous activity in man is unclear. One of the effects by which the alpha-2-agonist clonidine lowers blood pressure may be by stimulation of such peripheral receptors. In tetraplegics, hypertension following bladder stimulation is attenuated by pretreatment with clonidine (Mathias et al. 1979 a); these effects, however, may result from actions on sympathetic neurones in the spinal cord. There is experimental evidence to suggest that activation of peripheral alpha-2-receptors depends on much higher concentrations of clonidine than achieved clinically (Haeusler 1976). The availability of more specific alpha-2-adrenoreceptor antagonists and agonists may provide further information on the physiological function of these receptors.

Stimulation of presynaptic beta-adrenoceptors, on the other hand, results in the release of noradrenaline (Langer 1981). These receptors appear to be activated mainly by circulating adrenaline, which may also be taken up by the nerve terminal and released as a cotransmitter (Majewski et al. 1981). Some patients with essential hypertension have elevated levels of plasma adrenaline (Franco-Morselli et al. 1977). This may be 'stress' related and it has been hypothesized that in such patients the facilitatory effects of adrenaline may ultimately produce a sustained increase in sympathetic nervous activity, and hence hypertension (Brown and Macquin 1981). Secretion of adrenaline appears to be autonomous only in patients with phaeochromocytoma, and is otherwise probably centrally dependent as in tetraplegics we have found no change in plasma adrenaline levels in response to profound falls in blood pressure after hypoglycaemia or during activation of spinal sympathetic reflexes (Mathias et al. 1976, 1979 b and 1980). In patients with essential hypertension the difficulty in separating a selective increase in adrenaline, with its attendant peripheral presynaptic effects, from a nonselective central increase in sympathetic neuronal and adrenal activity remains both a conceptual and an experimental enigma.

Noradrenaline acts on postsynaptic receptors in target organs and these appear to be predominantly of the alpha-1-adrenoceptor subtype, especially those close to the nerve terminal. Stimulation of these innervated receptors causes smooth muscle contraction. The number of receptors and their affinity for noradrenaline are important in determining the target organ response. Several approaches have been used to study such receptors, including the use of radiologands. In man, because of limitations in obtaining vascular tissue, studies have been conducted on accessible cell membranes, such as the platelet (for alpha-adrenoceptor studies) and the lymphocyte (for beta-adrenoreceptor studies). The predominant receptor subtype varies on each cell. For instance, alpha-2-receptors predominate on platelets. This has raised questions about the validity of extrapolating such data to cardiovascular function. To overcome this problem some studies have combined pharmacological and biochemical responses. Patients with gross sympathetic failure, for example, exhibit exaggerated pressor responses to infused noradrenaline and have increased alpha-receptor binding sites on platelets (Davies et al. 1982). By contrast, tetraplegic patients who also have enhanced noradrenaline pressor sensitivity have normal platelet receptor numbers. This finding suggests that both increased receptor numbers and baroreceptor dysfunction account for the enhanced responses in patients with chronic autonomic failure while the latter alone is responsible in tetraplegics. Patients with essential hypertension also exhibit increased pressor responsiveness to infused noradrenaline (Philipp et al. 1978), but these patients also show impaired baroreflex sensitivity (Goldstein 1983), which make it difficult to dissect out the effects on receptors alone.

Studies of regional vascular responses to pharmacological agents have provided a further method of assessing postsynaptic receptor responsiveness. The vascular bed of the forearm lends itself to such studies in man. In patients with essential hypertension, alpha-1-receptor antagonists, such as prazosin cause a greater increase in forearm blood flow than the non-specific vasodilator nitroprusside; this is interpreted as representing enhanced postsynaptic alpha-adrenoreceptor activity in essential hypertension (Bolli et al. 1981). Whether the response in this particular vascular bed is representative of a true generalized defect in such patients is not known.

Target organ responses: the kidney

The sympathetic nervous system acts on a number of organs, and their responses may subsequently influence blood pressure. A prime example is the kidney. Sympathetic activation can alter renal haemodynamics, the release of renin, or the tubular absorption of sodium – and each may directly or indirectly influence blood pressure (Peart 1978; Gottschalk 1979). Angiotensin II, for instance, affects blood pressure by a number of mechanisms. It is directly vasopressor; it stimulates aldosterone secretion, which causes salt and water retention, plasma volume expansion and enhanced pressor responsiveness; and it also interacts with the sympathetic nervous system, both centrally and peripherally. The central sympathetic effects of angiotensin II in raising blood pressure have been clearly documented in animals (Ferrario 1983) and there is evidence that in man they may contribute to the maintenance of hypertension in patients with renal artery stenosis (Mathias et al. 1983).

Angiotensin II also has peripheral influences on the sympathetic neuroeffector junction. It may enhance release, decrease uptake, or diminish clearance of noradrenaline from the synaptic site (Zimmerman, 1981). It is one of many substances, including prostaglandins, calcium, sodium and potassium which can influence sympathetic nervous function. It is likely that a large number of peptides will be added to this list (Hokfelt et al. 1980). This may be of particular importance in the gastrointestinal tract, which has a rich and varied supply of peptides close to the largest vascular bed, the splanchnic circulation.

Blood pressure control

The effect on blood pressure, of activation of the peripheral sympathetic nervous system therefore depends on a number of factors; afferent pathways, cerebral centres, spinal outflow, peripheral sympathetic nerves, the state of the effector organs and their local milieu. The final effects vary in different vascular beds and in diverse situations. Normal responses clearly depend on integration of the entire system, and this is apparent in patients with either neural lesions or biochemical disorders which affect blood pressure. This may be of relevance to patients with essential hypertension who could have occult central or peripheral lesions. The availability of highly specific pharmacological agents, and the ability to study patients with clearly defined disorders, some without complex reflex effects, should now enable us to further unravel the intricate mechanisms involved in blood pressure control. This information should lead us to more rational and effective treatment of hypertensive patients and hopefully to the mechanisms which cause 'essential hypertension'.

Acknowledgements

I would like to thank Miss Joanne Coughtrey for her help with this manuscript and the Wellcome Trust for a Senior Wellcome Fellowship in Clinical Science.

29

References

1 Bolli P, Amann FW, Hulthen L, Kiowski W, Bühler FR (1981) Elevated plasma adrenaline reflects sympathetic overactivity and enhanced α-adrenoreceptor-mediated vasoconstriction in essential hypertension. Clin Sci 61:161s–164s.

2 Brod J, Fencl V, Hejl Z, Jirka J (1959) Circulatory changes underlying blood pressure elevation during acute emotional stress (mental arithmetic) in normotensive and hypertensive subjects. Clin Sci 18:269–279.

3 Brown MJ, Macquin I (1981) Is adrenaline the cause of essential hypertension? Lancet ii:1079–1082.

4 Corbett JL, Frankel HL, Harris PJ (1971) Cardiovascular reflex reponses to cutaneous and visceral stimulation in spinal man. J Physiol 215:395–401.

5 da Costa DF, Mathias CJ, Peart WS (unpublished results).

6 Davies IB, Mathias CJ, Sudera D, Sever PS (1982) Agonist regulation of alpha-adrenergic receptor responses in man. J Cardiovasc Pharmacol 4:s139–s144.

7 Ferrario CM (1983) Central nervous system mechanisms of blood pressure control in normotensive and hypertensive states. Chest 83 (Suppl 2):331–335.

8 Franco-Morselli R, Elghozi JL, Joly E, di Giulio S, Meyer P (1977) Increased plasma adrenaline concentrations in benign essential hypertension. Br Med J ii:1251–1254.

9 Goldstein DS (1983) Arterial baroreflex sensitivity, plasma catecholamines, and pressor responsiveness in essential hypertension. Circulation 68:234–240.

10 Gottschalk CW (1979) Renal nerves and sodium excretion. Ann Rev Physiol 41:229–240.

11 Haeusler G (1976) Studies on the possible contribution of a peripheral presynaptic action of clonidine and dopamine to their vascular effects under *in vivo* conditions. Naunyn-Schmiedeberg's Arch Pharmacol 295:191–202.

12 Hokfelt T, Johansson O, Ljungdahl A, Lundberg JM, Schultzberg M (1980) Peptidergic neurones. Nature 284:515–521.

13 Langer SZ (1981) Presynaptic regulation of the release of catecholamines. Pharmacol Rev 32:337–362.

14 Lewis T (1932) Vasovagal syncope and the carotid sinus mechanism. Br Med J 1:873–876.

15 Majewski H, Rand MJ, Tung LH (1981) Activation of prejunctional β-adrenoreceptors in rat atria by adrenaline applied exogenously or released as a cotransmitter. Br J Pharmacol 73:669–679.

16 Mathias CJ, Christensen NJ, Corbett JL, Frankel HL, Spalding JMK (1976) Plasma catecholamines during paroxysmal neurogenic hypertension in quadriplegic man. Circ Res 39:204–208.

17 Mathias CJ, Reid JL, Wing LMH, Frankel HL, Christensen NJ (1979a) Antihypertensive effects of clonidine in tetraplegic subjects devoid of central sympathetic control. Clin Sci Molec Med 57:425s–428s.

18 Mathias CJ, Frankel HL, Turner RC, Christensen NJ (1979b) Physiological responses to insulin hypoglycaemia in spinal man. Paraplegia 17:319–326.

19 Mathias CJ, Christensen NJ, Frankel HL, Peart WS (1980) Renin release during head-up tilt occurs independently of sympathetic nervous activity in tetraplegic man. Clin Sci 59:251–256.

20 Mathias CJ, Wilkinson A, Lewis PS, Peart WS, Sever PS, Snell ME (1983) Clonidine lowers blood pressure independently of renin suppression in patients with unilateral renal artery stenosis. Chest 83:(Suppl 2) 357–359.

21 Mathias CJ, Frankel HL (1983) Autonomic failure in tetraplegia. In: Bannister R (ed.) Autonomic failure: a textbook of clinical disorders of the autonomic nervous system. Oxford University Press, Oxford: 453–488.

22 Peart WS (1978) Intra-renal factors in renin release. Contrib Nephrol 12:5–15.

23 Philipp T, Distler A, Cordes U (1978) Sympathetic nervous system and blood pressure control in essential hypertension. Lancet ii:959–963.

24 Pickering TG, Bruckner B, Frankel HL, Mathias CJ, Dworkin BR, Miller NE (1977) Mechanisms of learned voluntary control of blood pressure in patients with generalized bodily paralysis. In: Beatty J and Legwie H (eds). Biofeedback and Behaviour, NATO Conference Series, Series III, Human Factors. Vol. 2, Plenum Press, New York, Section 3:225–234.

25 Reid JL, Wing LMH, Mathias CJ, Frankel HL, Neill E (1977) The central hypotensive effect of clonidine: studies in tetraplegic subjects. Clin Pharmacol Ther 21:375–381.
26 Smith AD (1973) Mechanisms involved in the release of noradrenaline from sympathetic nerves. Br Med Bull 29:123–129.
27 Weinshilboum RM, Thoa NB, Johnson DG, Kopin IJ, Axelrod J (1971) Proportional release of norepinephrine and dopamine-β-hydroxylase from sympathetic nerves. Science 174:1349–1351.
28 Weinshilboum RM (1983) Biochemical genetics of catecholamines in humans. Mayo Clin Proc 58:319–330.
29 Wing LMH, Reid JL, Hamilton CA, Sever P, Davies DS, Dollery CT (1977) Effects of clonidine on biochemical indices of sympathetic function and plasma renin activity in normotensive man. Clin Sci Molec Med 53:45–53.
30 Zimmerman BG (1981) Adrenergic facilitation by angiotensin; does it serve a physiological function? Clin Sci 60:343–348.

Correspondence:
Dr. C. J. Mathias
Medical Unit,
St. Marys Hospital Medical School,
Norfolk Place,
London W2 18G
Great Britain

Discussion

MCMAHON:
Have you or anyone else studied the effects of ageing on the number of platelet alpha-receptors?

MATHIAS:
We have not. The numbers of beta-receptors and lymphocytes appear to decrease with age but I cannot recall platelet alpha-receptor studies in the elderly. They, of course, have raised plasma noradrenaline levels which appear to be secondary to diminished clearance rather than increased secretion. One might therefore expect platelet alpha-receptor numbers to be diminished although it is worth pointing out that there is no evidence of pressor hypersensitivity to alpha-agonists in the aged.

POLINSKY:
Have you found any relationship between either blood pressure or plasma noradrenaline and the level of transection in patients with tetraplegia?

MATHIAS:
Yes. Our colleague, Hans Frankel, studied blood pressure in a large group of spinal patients with transection at different levels and clearly observed that the higher the lesion the lower the blood pressure. We have not yet studied in a detailed manner the relationship between the level of the transection, blood pressure and plasma noradrenaline levels.

POLINSKY:
In your patients with complete transection there were no connections between the central and peripheral sympathetic pathways and I wondered whether the effect of clonidine, if it were a peripheral one, varied in relationship with the residual level or with plasma noradrenaline.

31

MATHIAS:

That is a possibility. The reason for studying the patients with high cervical transections is that they appear not to have connections between central control mechanisms and the peripheral sympathetic nervous system. We are reasonably sure that in the basal state (and this is borne out by the low levels of plasma noradrenaline) there is minimal sympathetic nervous activity and hence clonidine has no further effects in lowering blood pressure. I quite agree that the patients can very readily activate their spinal sympathetic outflow and the resultant elevation in blood pressure caused by this can be prevented by clonidine.

MANCIA:

Could you tell me your interpretation of the fall in blood pressure induced by clonidine in patients with renal artery stenosis?

MATHIAS:

We can substantially lower blood pressure in such patients in the absence of change in circulating levels of plasma renin activity and angiotensin II. A series of further studies, in progress, seems to indicate that there is no peripheral interaction between clonidine and other vasopressor substances. The pressor dose reponses to infused angiotensin II and to noradrenaline, for instance, are not diminished, making it very likely that the observed effects of clonidine in lowering blood pressure in our patients are exerted centrally. The raised blood pressure in renal artery stenosis patients therefore appears to be maintained by central nervous pressor mechanisms but this may not occur in the initial phase.

MANCIA:

I am surprised that renin secretion (if we equate plasma renin levels to renin secretion) is the same before and after clonidine in renal artery stenosis, because of the animal evidence that the sympathetic control of renin is also exerted by playing a permissive role over the renal baroreceptor and macula densa mechanisms. In animals, if you produce renal artery stenosis you get much more renin out of the innervated than the denervated kidney. So I would expect to see renin come down when you give a drug which reduces sympathetic control of the kidney.

MATHIAS:

We are not surprised at all. Professor Peart and I have been engaged in these studies for some time. We initially studied tetraplegics (who provided the initial evidence) in whom without activating the sympathetic nervous system you can cause a marked increase in circulating levels of renin. The key factor in them appears to be changes in blood pressure and renal perfusion pressure. It is likely that in our patients with renal artery stenosis the sympathetic nervous system is overridden by vascular changes resulting from ischaemia within the kidney; this probably maintains renin secretion (as in the tetraplegics) but is independent of sympathetic nervous activity.

MANCIA:

I see the difference but I wanted to emphasize the clear-cut contrast between human and animal studies. In animals if you produce acute renal hypertension and stimulate the renal nerves at a very low frequency (a fraction of a Hertz – which normally does not of itself change renin levels) there is a much greater increase in plasma renin. This is the difference with animal studies.

MATHIAS:

This is maybe why one should study man!

PEART:

It is a chronic preparation that we are studying in man. I have to remind you of early studies by Goldblatt and his colleagues. They studied renal artery stenosis acutaly in dogs; they raised blood pressure when they changed the blood flow to the kidney but a fact that people have forgotten was that they showed that yohimbine, given to the animals later on, when they had had hypertension due to renal artery stenosis for 6 weeks, lowered the blood pressure. This was at a time when its actions were not fully understood. Yohimbine did not lower the blood pressure in the acute stage but did so later on, and these are very old studies – 40 years old. These observations are now more relevant to man. Therefore what is interesting, I think, is that maybe the central nervous system is taking a much greater part in maintaining blood pressure in these later stages than certainly I had ever thought.

HAYDUK:
Do you have any idea of the response to peripherally acting drugs like nifedipine, hydralazine or captopril in these tetraplegic patients? Is there a normal or changed response?

MATHIAS:
The quick answer is that drugs which act directly on blood vessels produce a greater fall in blood pressure in tetraplegics than in normal subjects. This appears to be related to their being unable to increase compensatory sympathetic activity.

MCMAHON:
Were these renal artery stenosis patients an homogeneous population? Were they bilateral or unilateral?

MATHIAS:
In the data presented all 9 patients had unilateral renal artery stenosis, which was due to either fibromuscular hyperplasia or atheroma.

MACMAHON:
Did you use converting enzyme inhibitors?

MATHIAS:
We did study the effects of converting enzyme inhibitors but mainly in response to a single dose. In some of the patients, but not all, there was a fall in blood pressure.

WEBER:
What would happen if you first gave a converting enzyme inhibitor and then administered clonidine? Would it still have an antihypertensive effect?

MATHIAS:
We do not know the answer to this question but it would be of considerable interest.

WEBER:
This has been studied in animals by Dr Oparil and her group in Alabama; she claims that there are two separate mechanisms involved.

SAMBHI:
Some years ago we looked at the effect of oral clonidine treatment on renin levels in patients with essential hypertension. Patients with a low plasma renin activity had a slight rise in renin and those with a higher renin activity had a slight fall. In our hands, therefore, clonidine does not necessarily suppress plasma renin activity. A quick question to Dr Mathias. You have shown that clonidine, while it changed noradrenaline levels and blood pressure, had no effect on adrenaline in tetraplegic patients, but your tetraplegics showed rather low levels of adrenaline.

MATHIAS:
They do indeed, but interpreting adrenaline levels is difficult because of the extremely low levels normally seen. These are close to the limits of the assay sensitivity. There is no doubt, however, that the levels of adrenaline in the tetraplegics were lower than in normal subjects and did not change after clonidine.

Baroreflex function and centrally acting antihypertensive drugs

G. P. Guthrie, Jr.

The baroreflex is a neural circuit that has powerful effects on blood pressure and heart rate. First recognized in the 1920s (Koch and Mies 1929), it is now known to involve sensory endings (arterial baroreceptors) in both the carotid sinus and the aortic arch. These produce afferent impulses which are transmitted via the glossopharyngeal (carotid) and vagus (aortic) nerves to synapses within the nucleus tractus solitarius of the medulla. Ultimately, blood pressure and heart rate are affected by parallel sympathetic and parasympathetic modulation. Following the initial description of the baroreflex, it was speculated that a primary disturbance of its function might lead to hypertension in man. This speculation remains active today, supported by observations that impairment of the baroreflex function can produce hypertension in animals and in man. The development of centrally acting antihypertensive drugs, including clonidine hydrochloride, has provided further information about the neurophysiology of the baroreflex, including evidence that baroreflex modulation may be a component action of such drugs.

Baroreflex and arterial pressure

Following the original descriptions of the carotid sinus reflex, experiments were carried out in the 1930s and 1940s to examine the effects of peripheral denervation of carotid and aortic baroreceptors (Nowak 1940). They supported the initial speculation that impairment of the baroreflex might lead to hypertension. Animals with virtual abolition of all baroreflex function developed a neurogenic type of hypertension characterized by tachycardia and labile and occasionally extreme blood pressure elevations. More recent experiments with sinoaortic denervated dogs have shown elevations of mean blood pressure which are less pronounced (Cowley et al. 1973). Only moderate, labile blood pressure elevations (about 12 mm Hg in mean arterial pressure) have been noted. This latter factor is reflected by a widening of the 24-hour frequency distribution curves for blood pressure (Fig. 1), which suggests that the predominant function of the baroreflex is to minimize variations in arterial blood pressure rather than its set point. However, modest elevations of mean blood pressure did occur in these more recent studies, despite the artificial environment of the animals, which shielded them from normal, minimal environmental stresses.

In man, less radical interference with baroreflex function than described above leads to either labile or sustained hypertension. Neurosurgeons have long recognized that severance of a single glossopharyngeal nerve (carrying carotid sinus afferents) in the treatment of glossopharyngeal tic syndrome leads to labile hypertension and tachycardia. Several reports note sustained hypertension in main after this and similar procedures (Ripley et al. 1977; Sleight 1979).

34

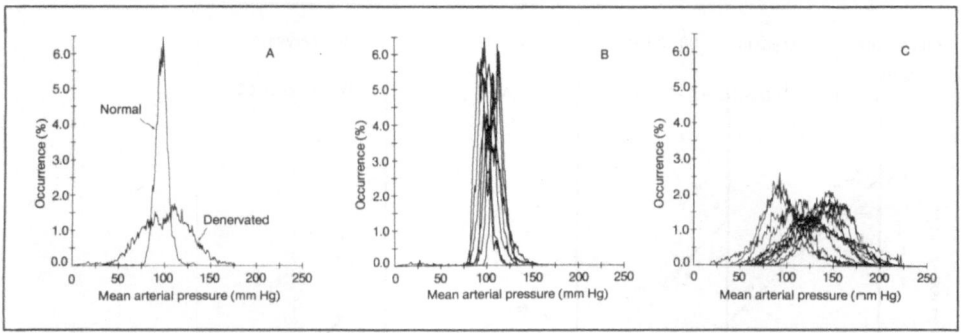

Fig. 1. Frequency distribution curves of 24-hour continuous recordings of mean arterial blood pressure in both normal and sinoaortic denervated dogs. (A): An individual dog before and after denervation. (B): A composite overlay of 10 normal dogs. (C): A composite overlay of 12 denervated dogs (Cowley at al. 1973, by permission of the American Heart Association, Inc.)

Most studies of baroreflex function in humans have used one of two techniques:
- measurement of the slowing of heart rate during injection of pressor agents such as phenylephrine;
- measurement of changes in blood pressure of heart rate in response to stimulation of the carotid sinus by neck suction.

Each technique has disadvantages, such as the reliance of the pressor hormone method on heart rate changes alone, and the inability of the neck chamber method to affect aortic arch baroreceptors.

In the 1960s, Smyth and co-workers (1969) used phenylephrine injections to study the impairment of baroreflex function in several forms of human hypertension. Their results, which have been confirmed in subsequent studies (Korner et al. 1974; Takeshita et al. 1975; Simon et al. 1977), show that patients with sustained essential hypertension have diminished baroreflex control of heart rate compared with agematched normotensive individuals (baroreflex sensitivity also normally diminishes with age) (Gribbin et al. 1971) (Fig. 2). Others have found similar results with the neck chamber technique confirming that diminished baroreflex sensitivity appears to be a common abnormality following sustained elevation of the blood pressure. Investigations by Takishita and co-workers (1975) and Eckberg (1979) have shown that reduced baroreceptor sensitivity is an early abnormality in hypertension. Diminished sensitivity is found in patients with borderline forms of the disease in comparison with age-matched normal subjects. Takishita found that nine nineteen-year-old patients with borderline hypertension averaged baroreceptor slopes of 9.1 msec/mm Hg, compared with average slopes of 16 msec/mm Hg in six normotensive sujects of comparable age (Fig. 3).

Eckberg found further evidence of a gradation of baroreflex responsiveness among patients classified as having borderline hypertension. Significantly reduced responsiveness occurred only in those subjects whose average systolic blood pressures were greater than 140 mm Hg. Suggestive but non-significant impairment of the baroreflex was seen in borderline hypertensives with average systolic blood pressures less than 140 mm Hg.

35

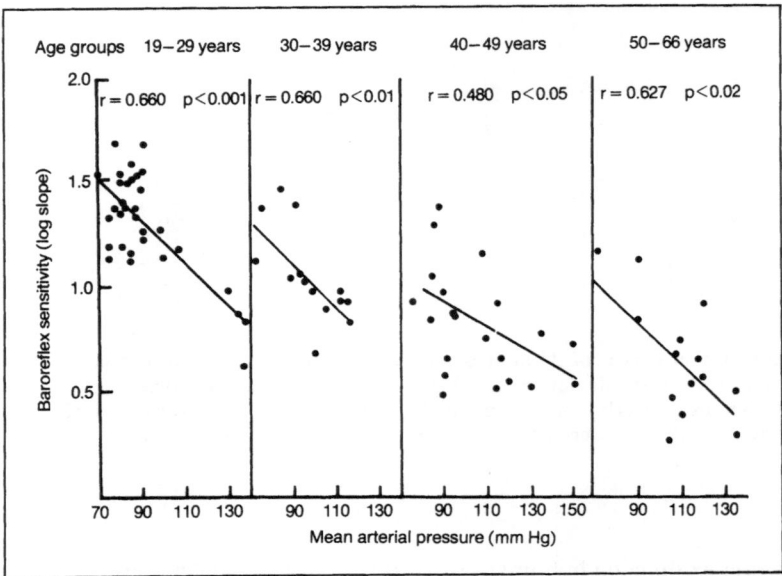

Fig. 2. Correlation of baroreflex sensitivity and the resting mean arterial pressure of patients with both normotension and hypertension. Subjects are divided into groups by age. (Gribbin et al. 1971, by permission of the American Heart Association, Inc.)

We have investigated baroreflex activity as a function of blood pressure in 23 young adult males from Bourbon County, Kentucky, an area with a high prevalence of hypertension (Kotchen et al. 1982). Assessing baroreflex slope via an indirect method using bolus phenylephrine injections, similar to that previously described by Smyth et al. (1969), we found that normotensive young adult males with similar blood pressures did not have differing baroreflex slopes. Since we presume that those with relatively high blood pressures (from the upper decile of the distribution) have an increased risk of later sustained hypertension, our findings imply that primary abnormalities of the baroreflex might not be involved in the genesis of hypertension. Data from the spontaneously hypertensive rat (Brown 1980) suggest that baroreflex is in fact reset by elevated arterial pressure. Resetting normally occurs in the early stages of hypertension, but it is eliminated if these rats are rendered normotensive from six weeks of age with drug therapy. Hence, from these studies, it seems likely that impairment of baroreflex function is the result of hypertension, although whether it might also be a cause of it remains an unanswered question. Since baroreceptor endings in both the carotid sinus and aortic arch are near the junction of the muscular media and adventitia of the artery (Sleight 1979), alterations in baroreflex function might be induced by vascular changes produced by hypertension, including thickening or decreased elasticity of the arterial wall.

Effect of antihypertensive drugs on the baroreflex

Central modulation of baroreflex function by antihypertensive drugs has been described in both animal and human forms of hypertension. Although the precise mecha-

36

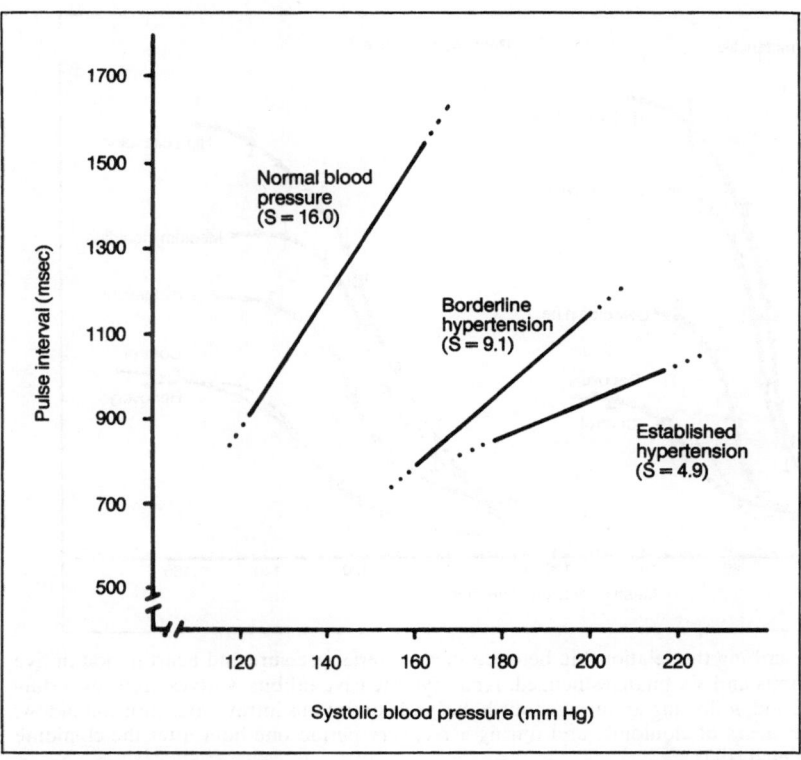

Fig. 3. Comparison of the linear regressions relating baroreceptor sensitivity after phenylephrine injections in six normal subjects, nine patients with borderline hypertension of the same age, and in 14 older patients with established essential hypertension. Mean slopes of the regressions (5, msec/mm Hg) differ significantly from each other (P < 001) (Takishita et al 1975, by permission of the American Heart Association, Inc.)

nism of the antihypertensive action of the beta-adrenergic blockers remains controversial, it is possible that they reduce blood pressure through interaction with the central nervous system. Early studies on the baroreflex in hypertensive man suggested that the beta-adrenergic blocker propranolol enhanced baroreflex sensitivity in normal subjects (Sleight et al. 1979). However, Simon et al. (1977b), failed to confirm an alteration in the baroreflex sensitivity of patients with essential hypertension after short-term or long-term treatment with either propranolol or timolol. Several studies have shown the potentiating effect of clonidine on the baroreflex. Clonidine is thought to act upon the nucleus tractus solitarius within the medulla, an important cardiovascular centre involved in the baroreflex loop. Aars (1972), Kobinger and Walland (1972) and Hausler (1977) have reported *in vivo* potentiation of baroreflex function in normotensive animals. Following intravenous clonidine, clear resetting of baroreflex sensitivity in both normal and renal hypertensive rabbits, together with blood pressure reductions in both models, have been described by Korner et al. (1975) (Fig. 4). Subsequently, Sleight and West (1975) reported that acute intravenous injection of clonidine potentiated the baroreflex heart rate at response by 48% in seven human subjects, two with borderline

37

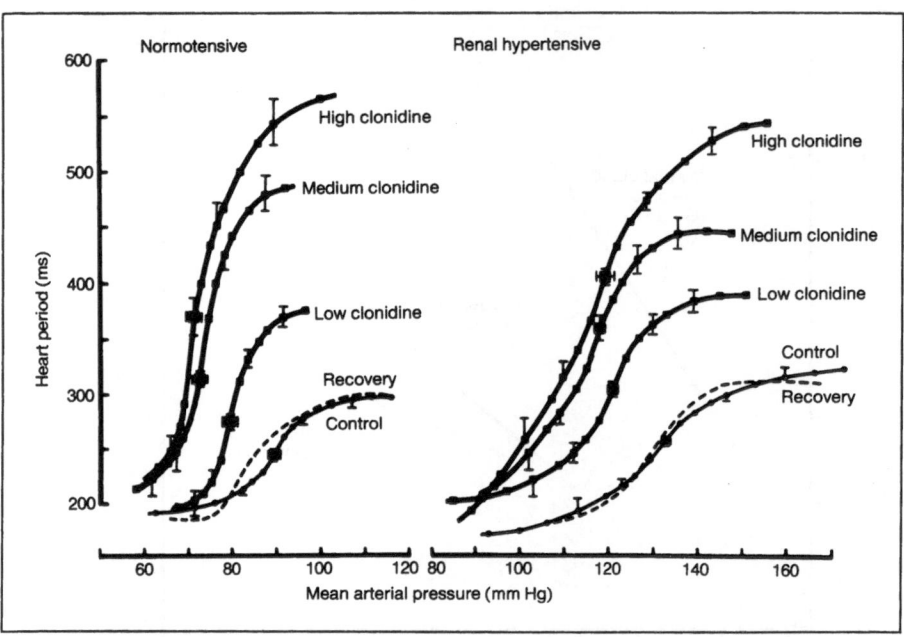

Fig. 4. Curves describing the relationship between mean arterial pressure and heart period in five normotensive rabbits and six unanaesthetized, renal hypertensive rabbits. Curves are shown during the control period, following an intravenous bolus and continuous intravenous infusion of low, medium and high doses of clonidine, and during a recovery period one hour after the clonidine infusion. (Korner et al. 1975)

hypertension. However, Mancia et al. (1979) found no significant effect of clonidine as detected by the neck chamber method. We assessed the effects of clonidine on the baroreflex in a group of 30 patients with mild to moderately severe hypertension (Guthrie and Kotchen 1983). Following three weeks of placebo treatment the baroreflex slope of patients was measured and they were then treated with oral clinidine in divided doses, ranging from 0.2–0.4 mg/day. This prescription was sufficient to reduce their diastolic blood pressures 10% below baseline for the subsequent six to eight weeks, after which they were restudied. Oral clonidine enhanced baroreflex sensitivity in 26 of 30 patients and significantly increased mean baroreflex slope by 78% (Fig. 5).

At the same time, plasma noradrenaline and adrenaline concentrations and heart rate were reduced and sensitivity to phenylephrine was increased. Our results, together with those previously cited, suggest that clonidine hydrochloride potentiates baroreflex function in both human and experimental hypertension. This potentiation might be a component (although not an obligate mechanism) for the antihypertensive action of the drug.

We have also investigated the effects of clonidine in patients with mild hypertension and adult onset type diabetes mellitus. Since many antihypertensive drugs carry the potential to effect glucose tolerance, we sought to assess both the effectiveness of clonidine for the treatment of mildly hypertensive diabetics and its effects on glucose metabolism and the baroreflex. We found that, as in non-diabetic hypertensives, clonidine in-

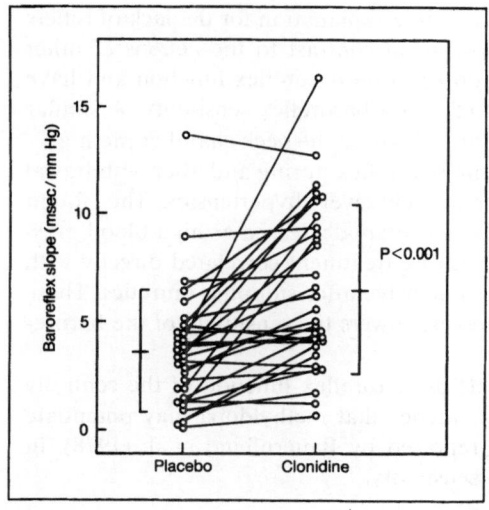

Fig. 5. Baroreflex slope during placebo treatment and after long-term oral clonidine therapy in 30 patients with essential hypertension. (Guthrie and Kotchen 1983)

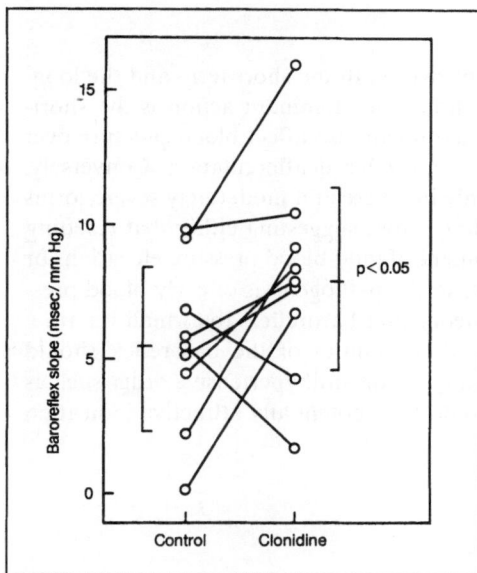

Fig. 6. Baroreflex slope in nine patients with both mild hypertension and adult onset type diabetes mellitus before and after sustained oral clonidine treatment. (Guthrie et al. 1983)

creased baroreflex slope in seven out of nine patients with a mean increment of 44% (Fig. 6). Clonidine also significantly increased the incremental area under the intravenous glucose tolerance curve, but did not significantly affect diabetic control, as reflected by levels of fasting serum glucose, urinary glucose excretion and glycohaemoglobin over the 10 weeks of treatment.

Other antihypertensive drugs have been less well studied for their effects on baroreflex function. Sasso and O'Connor (1982) reported that the peripherally acting alpha-adrenergic blocker, prazosin, depresses baroreflex sensitivity rather than enhances it.

These authors have suggested this effect as a possible explanation for the lack of reflelx tachycardia and hyper-reninaemia after prazosin, in contrast to the actions of other vasodilators. We have studied the effects of prazosin on baroreflex function and have noted that our methods show no significant effect on baroreflex sensitivity. A similar result has been obtained by Mancia et al. (1980), who used the neck chamber method.

Caretta and co-workers (1983) have studied the baroreflex during and after withdrawal of diuretic therapy in patients with mild to moderately severe hypertension. They found that after the cessation of diuretics, baroreflex sensitivity decreased as high blood pressure recurred, and that baroreflex sensitivity during treatment correlated directly with the time during which patients remained normotensive after stopping diuretics. These data support the idea that elevated blood pressure lowers the sensitivity of the baroreflex, rather than the converse.

Little work has been conducted on the effects on baroreflex function of the centrally active antihypertensive agent, methyldopa. Evidence that methyldopa may potentiate the baroreflex comes from a single patient reported by Bauernfeind et al. (1978), in whom this drug produced carotid sinus hypersensitivity.

Summary

The baroreflex undergoes important alterations over both the short-term and the long-term in animal and human hypertension. Although its dominant action is the short-term regulation of blood pressure, it is clear that it can also affect blood pressure over the long-term, as seen in complete or partial baroreflex deafferentation. Conversely, abnormalities in the baroreflex are seen not only in severe and moderately severe forms of hypertension, but also in mild and borderline states, suggesting either that resetting of baroreflex sensitivity is an early accompaniment of mild blood pressure elevations or that abnormalities in the baroreflex contribute to the pathogenesis of early blood pressure elevation. Most evidence supports the theory that baroreflex abnormalities are a secondary event. However, if mild primary abnormalities of the baroreflex should prove to be pathogenic, the capability of centrally acting antihypertensive drugs such as clonidine to potentiate baroreflex function would be a potentially attractive indication for their early use.

References

1 Aars H (1972) Effects of clonidine on aortic diameter and aortic baroreceptor activity. Eur J Pharmacol 20:52–59.
2 Bauernfeind R, Hall C, Denes P, Rosen KM (1978) Carotid sinus hypersensitivity with alpha methyldopa. Ann Int Med 88:214–215.
3 Brown AM (1980) Receptors under pressure: an update on baroreceptors. Circ Res 46:1–10.
4 Carretta R, Fabris B, Bellini G, Tonutti L, Battilana G, Bianchetti A, Campanacci L (1983) Baroreflex function after therapy withdrawal in patients with essential hypertension. Clin Sci 64:259–263.
5 Cowley AW Jr., Liard JF, Guyton AC (1973) Role of the baroreceptor reflex in daily control of arterial blood pressure and other variables in dogs. Circ Res 32:564–576.
6 Eckberg DL (1979) Carotid baroreflex function in young men with borderline blood pressure elevation Circulation 59:623–636.

7 Gribbin B, Pickering TG, Sleight P, Peto R (1971) Effect of age and high blood pressure on baroreflex sensitivity in man. Circ Res 29:424–431.
8 Guthrie GP Jr., Kotchen TA (1983) Effects of oral clonidine on baroreflex function in patients with essential hypertension. Chest 83 (Suppl):327–328.
9 Haeusler G (1977) Neuronal mechanisms influencing transmission in the baroreceptor reflex arc. In: De Jong W, Provoost SP, Shapiro AP (eds), Hypertension and Brain Mechanisms, Prog Brain Res 47:95–109.
10 Kobinger W, Walland A (1972) Evidence for a central activation of a vagalcardiodepressor reflex by clonidine. Eur J Pharmacol 19:203–209.
11 Koch E, Mies A (1929) Chronischer arterieller Hochdruck durch experimentelle Dauerausschaltung der Blutdruckzügler. Krankheitsforsch 7:241–256.
12 Korner PI, West MJ, Shaw J, Uther JB (1974) Steady state properties of the baroreceptor-heart rate reflex in essential hypertension in man. Clin Exp Pharmacol Physiol 1:65–76.
13 Korner PI, Oliver JR, Sleight P, Robinson JS, Chalmers JP (1975) Assessment of cardiac autonomic excitability in renal hypertensive rabbits using clonidine-induced resetting of the baroreceptor-heart rate reflex. Eur J Pharmacol 33:353–362.
14 Kotchen TA, Guthrie GP Jr., McKean H, Kotchen JM (1982) Adrenergic responsiveness in prehypertensive subjects. Circulation 65:285–290.
15 Mancia G, Ferrari A, Gregorini L, Zanchetti A (1979). Clonidine and carotid baroreflex in essential hypertension. Hypertension 1:362–370.
16 Mancia G, Ferrari A, Gregorini L, Ferrari C, Bianchini C, Terzoli L, Leonetti G, Zanchetti A (1980) Effect of prazosin on autonomic control of circulation in essential hypertension. Hypertension 2:700–707.
17 Nowak SJG (1940) Chronic hypertension produced by carotid sinus and aortic-depressor nerve section. Ann Surg 111:102–111.
18 Ripley RC, Hollifield JW, Nies AS (1977) Sustained hypertension after section of the glossopharyngeal nerve. Am J Med 62:297–302
19 Sasso EH, O'Connor DT (1982) Prazosin depression of baroreflex function in hypertensive man. Eur J Clin Pharmacol 22:7–14.
20 Simon AC, Safar ME, Weiss YA, London GM, Milliez PL (1977a) Baroreflex sensitivity and cardiopulmonary blood volume in normotensive and hypertensive patients. Br Heart J 39:799–805.
21. Simon G, Kiowski W, Julius S (1977b) Effect of beta-adrenoceptor antagonists on baroreceptor reflex sensitivity in hypertension Clin Pharmacol Ther 22:293–298.
22 Sleight P, West MJ (1975) The effects of clonidine on the baroreflex arc in man. In: Davies DS, Reid JL (eds). Central action of drugs in blood pressure regulation. Pitman Medical, Tunbridge, Wells 291–299.
23 Sleight P (1979) Reflex control of the heart. AM J Cardio 44:889–894.
24 Sleight P, Gribbin B, Pickering TG (1979) Baroreflex sensitivity in normal and hypertensive man: the effect of beta adrenergic blockade on reflex sensitivity. Post Grad Med J 47:79–81.
25 Smyth HS, Sleight P, Pickering GW (1969) Reflex regulation of arterial pressure during sleep in man: a quantitative method of assessing baroreflex sensitivity. Circ Res 24:109–112.
26 Takeshita et al. (1975) Circulation 51:739.

Correspondence:
Gordon P. Guthrie JR., M.D.
Division of Endocrinology
Department of Medicine
University of Kentucky College of Medicine
Lexington, KY 40536, USA

Discussion

TUCK:
Was there any difference in basic baroreceptor function between diabetic and nondiabetic hypertensives?

GUTHRIE:
No, they were comparable to our hypertensive controls.

TUCK:
What dose of clonidine did you give these subjects?

GUTHRIE:
It was the same dose, 0.1–0.2 mg, no higher, over 10 weeks of treatment.

POLINSKY:
Was there anything special about the three diabetic hypertensives whose blood pressure seemed to go in the opposite direction to the rest of the group? Did they have diabetic neuropathies?

GUTHRIE:
No patients had neuropathy. We carefully selected patients without end organ damage using conventional criteria, and there was nothing to distinguish them from the others in terms of their blood pressure response or example.

PEART:
Are you surprised by the results of denervation experiments in man? Do you think you should take account of the carotid body? If that is denervated, or destroyed, there is no doubt that the patients develop respiratory abnormalities in the early stages; some become almost apnoeic for a while after this operation.
Are you even more surprised that you get a change in blood pressure by devervation of one side only?

GUTHRIE:
I am surprised that if one of four afferent trunks is severed there are such pronounced changes in blood pressure.

PEART:
Yes, and so therefore I suspect the specificity of what is being described.

Haemodynamic effects of antihypertensive agents in man

G. Mancia and A. Zanchetti

The haemodynamic effects of drugs affecting the neutral control of blood pressure in humans can be considered from various standpoints. A long list could be produced of antihypertensive agents acting wholly or partly through the sympathetic nervous system. It would include some drugs not formerly recognized as being in this category (e.g. the diuretics and perhaps even the calcium antagonists). Such drugs cause changes in the peripheral circulation and in the neuromodulation of hormones (such as renin and antidiuretic hormone) which are important in the control of blood pressure and blood volume. The relationship between the clinical effects of these drugs in man and their modes and sites of action in animals is also a matter of considerable interest. This paper, however, concentrates on the effects of antihypertensive drugs on neural cardiovascular regulation and blood pressure homoeostasis.

The development and use of drugs affecting the sympathetic nervous system has constituted a major approach to antihypertensive treatment. Towards the end of the 1940s the first serious attempt to treat severe and malignant hypertension involved the use of ganglion-blocking agents, but these proved unacceptable because they reduced cardiac output and, more importantly, caused hypotension and collapse in the upright posture and during exercise. Hence, such antisympathetic drugs, while reducing vasoconstrictor activity and high blood pressure, were of limited value because of interference with normal cardiovascular homoeostasis. Similar but less pronounced problems were experienced by patients taking alpha-blockers, such as phentolamine or sympatholytic agents such as guanethidine.

However, the idea that drugs which reduce blood pressure through interference with the sympathetic system inevitably disturb blood pressure homoeostasis has been proved erroneous by the development of drugs (i.e. methyldopa and clonidine) with a central, rather than a peripheral, site of action. Methyldopa has been shown to cause pronounced hypotension in patients in a supine position (1). Cardiac output was unaffected in these patients, so that the entire effect was attributable to a reduction in peripheral resistance. This is highly desirable in an antihypertensive drug, since hypertension reflects an abnormality of resistance and not one of cardiac output, at least in the established phase. In the same patients, the haemodynamic effects of dynamic exercise, isometric exercise, and exposure to cold were not affected by methyldopa treatment. Thus it could be concluded that haemodynamic responses to sympathetic activation were preserved despite the reduction in blood pressure and the vasodilation methyldopa had produced. We have found similar results with clonidine.

A fundamental mechanism of blood pressure control appears to involve arterial baroreflexes. It has been hypothesized that some antihypertensive agents working through the sympathetic system may impair baroreflexes by reducing the ability of sympathetic traffic to charge (or of noradrenaline to be discharged in response to alterations of the baroreceptor signal) the nerve terminals.

Animal experiments have shown some of the effects of impaired baroreflexes. Sino-aortic nerve section in an unrestrained, unanaesthetized cat, for instance, produces sharp fluctuations in blood pressure (2). Thus, impairment of baroreflexes may lead to blood pressure lability and, of course, this may be particularly undesirable in hypertension.

Some properties of sympatholytic drugs may, however, enhance the baroreceptor control of circulation. Korner et al. (3) studied the reflex changes in the R-R interval in unanaesthetized rabbits when the mean arterial pressure was reduced by deflating a cuff around the inferior vena cava, or increased by inflating a cuff around the thoracic aorta. The ability of the reflex to moderate the heart rate was greatly increased by several doses of clonidine. It was suggested that the enhancement of the baroreflex by clonidine was the mechanism involved in the hypotensive effect of the drug. A parallel hypothesis has been advanced to explain the hypotensive action of some betablockers (4).

In humans, the baroreceptor vagal heart rate reflex can be readily evoked by vasoactive drugs (5). This approach, however, leaves unexplored the main function of the arterial baroreflex which is the modulation of blood pressure by baroreceptors via changes in sympathetic activity. The control of blood pressure and modulation of sympathetic activity is difficult to study but we have developed a technique which uses a variable pressure neck chamber (6). A collar is placed on the patient's neck and decreasing or increasing pneumatic pressure can be applied. When a negative pressure is applied, the carotid transmural pressure rises, carotid baroreceptors are activated, and there is a reflex fall in blood pressure. The reverse happens if a positive pressure is applied (i.e. there is a reduction in the activity of the carotid baroreceptors and the blood pressure rises).

We have studied the baroreceptor control of blood pressure in normotensive controls, in subjects with moderate essential hypertension, and in subjects with severe essential hypertension (7, 8). The pressor response to reduction in carotid transmural pressure was smallest in those with severe essential hypertension and largest in the normotensive controls. The depressor response to baroreceptor stimulation, however, was smallest in the normotensive subjects and greatest in the hypertensive subjects. These data, and similar results from animal studies (9, 10) suggest that the baroreflex sensitivity is not altered in hypertension and that the early concept that associated this condition with an impairment of such reflex only pertains to its vagal modulatory ability. Blood pressure control seems to be largely preserved in hypertension. The opposite changes in pressor and depressor response can be explained on the basis of a marked resetting of the baroreflex. The assumption can be made that the set point of the reflex moves, not towards saturation, as would be expected when blood pressure rises, but towards threshold. Thus, in hypertension, the blood pressure is higher but the reflex is basically less stimulated, while retaining the ability to produce changes in blood pressure. This means a marked or exaggerated resetting of the baroreflex.

With regard to the influence of centrally-acting drugs on the baroreceptor control of blood pressure, our observations have shown that, during methyldopa treatment,

44

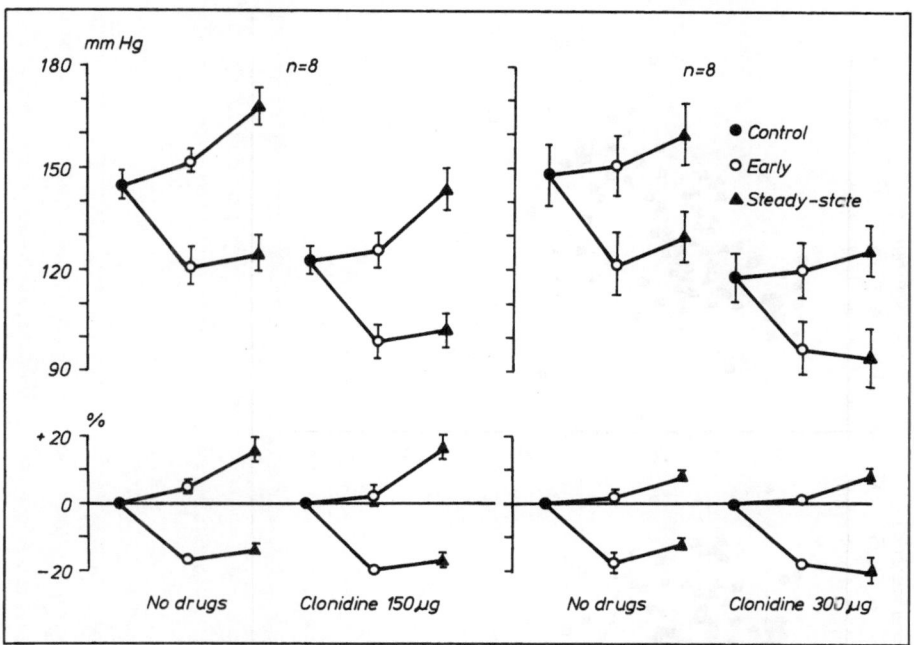

Fig. 1. Pressor and depressor responses to carotid baroreceptor deactivation and stimulation respectively before and after clonidine. Black circles refer to control values, and white circles and triangles to early and sustained responses to the baroreceptor manipulation. Percent. responses are shown at the bottom. (From Mancia et al., Hypertension 1:362 (1979), by permission.)

depressor responses to baroreceptor stimulation were virtually unaffected, whereas pressor responses to baroreceptor deprivation are only slightly reduced (1).

In one series of observations (11), we studied eight subjects before and after intravenous administration of 150 µg clonidine. Fig. 2 (left panel) shows baseline blood pressures before and after clonidine together with the pressor responses to baroreceptor deactivation, and the depressor responses to baroreceptor stimulation. The responses are identical before and after the drug, despite the hypotension produced by it. In another eight patients (Fig. 1, right panel) the dose of clonidine was 300 µg, causing an even greater hypotension, and the pressor and depressor responses to the baroreceptor manipulation were similarly unaffected. Thus clonidine neither impairs nor potentiates baroreceptor control of blood pressure and there seem to be no grounds for thinking that its clinical effect depends on involvement of this reflex mechanism. The absence of change in the pressor and depressor responses, first at high blood pressure and then at the lower blood pressure produced by the drug, implies a rapid reversal of the resetting of the baroreflex. This may favour the maintenance of the hypertensive effect. It may also suggest that the factor responsible for the resetting of the baroreflex in hypertension has a strong functional, rather than an anatomical, component.

Is this functional resetting component specifically affected by clonidine, or is the effect nonspecific? There have been many demonstrations that baroreflexes can be

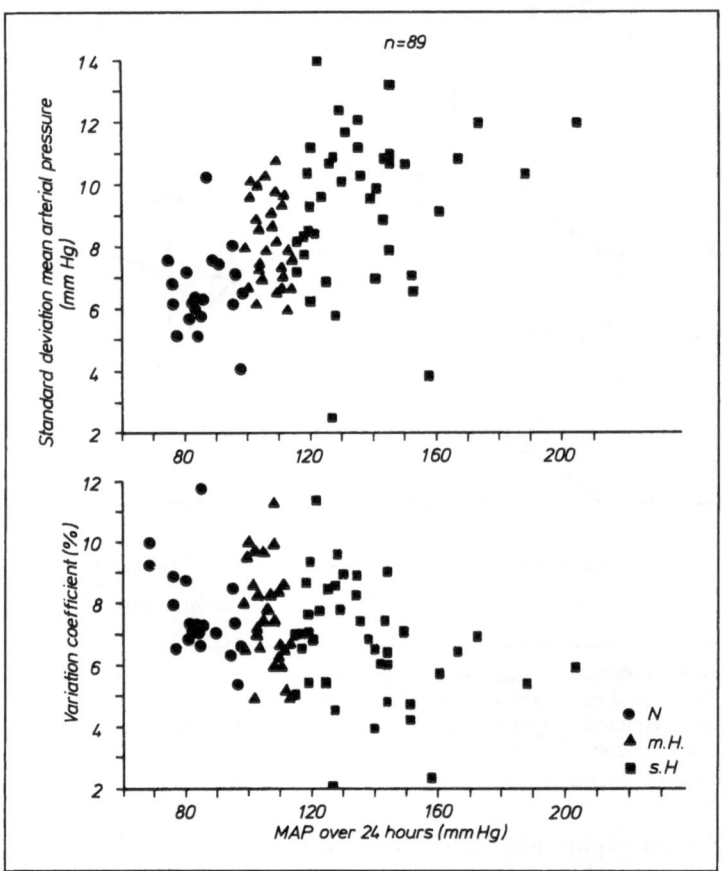

Fig. 2. Data from 89 ambulatory subjects in whom 24-hour mean arterial pressure (MAP) was recorded intra-arterially by means of the Oxford method. Symbols refer to the average MAP value throughout the 24 hours. The 24-hour absolute and percent. short-term MAP variability are plotted.

N: normotensives; m. H. and s. H.: moderate and severe hypertensives.

reset centrally (12). However, we have observed resetting not only with centrally-acting drugs like clonidine and methyldopa, but also with other drugs, some acting peripherally via different mechanisms (e.g. captopril, prazosin and beta-blockers) (4, 13, 14). The reversal of resetting is therefore more likely to be due to a nonspecific effect of the fall in blood pressure, irrespective of the mechanism reducing pressure. These data have helped to shape the current view of the ability of the baroreflex to adjust rapidly to whatever level is dictated by outside influences. This differs considerably from the old concept and limits the function of the baroreflex to that of defending perhaps only against short-term blood pressure variations, yielding whenever blood pressure changes are somewhat more persistent.

This may be why blood-pressure variability does not differ greatly between subjects with different blood pressure levels. Fig. 2 represents data from 89 ambulatory subjects

46

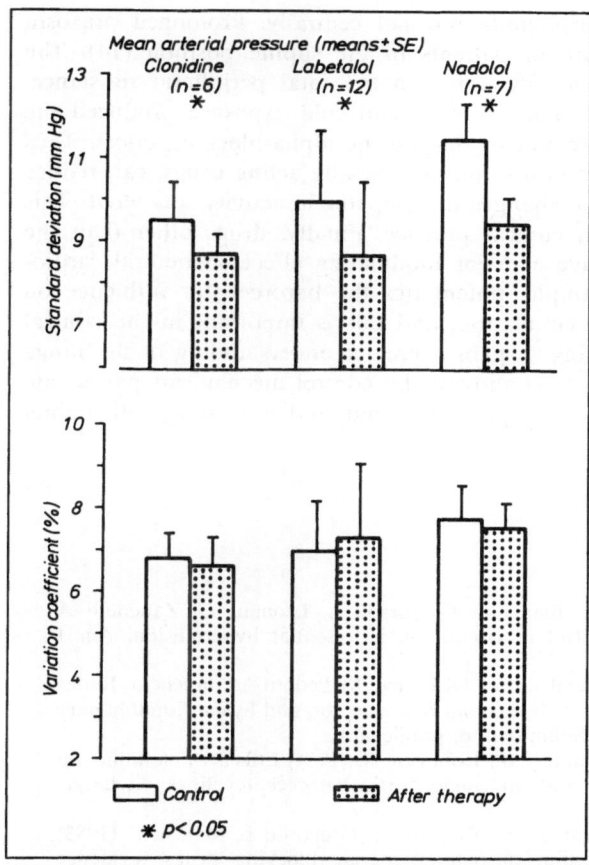

Fig. 3. Absolute and percent. short-term mean arterial pressure variability before and after antihypertensive treatment. (From Mancia, Chest 83:317 S (1983) by permission.)

in whom we recorded the intra-arterial blood pressure. Twenty-four hour mean arterial pressure variance was obtained together with the short-term standard variation and variation coefficient (averages of the 48 standard deviations and variation coefficients obtained separately for the 48 half hours of the recording). The standard deviation for mean arterial pressure tended to be higher in hypertensive than in normotensive subjects, but when baseline differences were allowed for an variability was expressed as variation coefficient, this tendency disappeared. Percentage blood pressure variations were similar over a wide range of mean 24-hour arterial pressure values.

A comparable result was obtained when the subjects were studied by the same technique before and after drug treatment. Fig. 3 shows results from three groups of subjects in whom blood pressure was recorded before and after treatment for about 2 weeks with clonidine, labetalol or nadolol. The standard deviation fell significantly, but the variation coefficient was unchanged, since the decrease was proportional to the reduction in pressure (15).

Prazosin is a drug which acts peripherally but not centrally. Prolonged prazosin therapy reduced the blood pressure of patients in the supine position (14). The reduction was entirely accounted for by a fall in the total peripheral resistance. Activation of the sympathetic system by exercise and cold exposure produced the same responses before and after treatment, despite the alpha-blocking effect. Thus not only centrally acting drugs, but also some peripherally acting drugs, can reduce the tonic level and leave the phasic changes in sympathetic activity unaltered. This property is of great importance in clinical practice. Finally, drugs other than the antihypertensive ones may also have a major modulating effect on neutral cardiovascular control. Digitalis, for example, potentiates the baroreceptor influence on both the heart and the peripheral circulation, and this is important in the clinical action of the drug (16, 17). Therefore to gain a greater understanding of the range and the extent to which alterations in cardiovascular control mechanisms participate in the effects of treatment it may be helpful to extend studies to drugs other than those with an antihypertensive effect.

References

1 Mancia G, Ferrari A, Gregorini L, Bianchini C, Terzoli L, Leonetti G, Zauchetti A (1980) Methyldopa and neural control of circulation in essential hypertension. Am J Cardiol 45:1237–1243.
2 Ramirez AJ, Bertinieri G, Belli L, Cavallazzi A, Di Rienzo M, Pedotti A, Mancia G: Reflex control of blood pressure and heart rate by arterial baroreceptor, and by cardiopulmonary receptors in the unanaesthetized cat. Submitted for publication.
3 Korner PI, Oliver JR, Sleight P, Chalmers JP, Robinson JS (1974) Effects of clonidine on the baroreceptor, heart rate reflex and on single aortic baroreceptor fibre discharge. Europ J Pharmacol 20:189–198.
4 Parati G, Pomidossi G, Grassi G, Gavazzi C, Ramirez A, Gregorini L, Mancia G (1983) Mechanisms of antihypertensive action of beta-adrenergic blocking drugs: evidence against potentiation of baroreflexes. Europ Heart J Suppl D, 4:19–25.
5 Bristow SD, Honour AS, Pickering GW, Sleight P, Smyth HS (1969) Diminished baroreflex sensitivity in high blood pressure. Circulation 39:48–54.
6 Ludbrook J, Mancia G, Ferrari A, Zauchetti A (1977) The variable pressure neck chamber method for studying the carotid baroreflex in man. Clin Sci Mol Med 53:165–172.
7 Mancia G, Ferrari A, Gregorini L, Valentini R, Ludbrook J, Zauchetti A (1977) Circulatory reflexes from carotid and extracarotid baroreceptor areas in man. Circulation Res 41:309–316.
8 Mancia G, Ludbrook J, Ferrari A, Gregorini L, Zauchetti A (1978) Baroreceptor reflexes in human hypertension. Circulation Res 43:170–177.
9 Ricksten Se, Thoan P (1981) Reflex control of sympathetic nerve activity and heart rate from arterial baroreceptors in conscious normotensive and spontaneously hypertensive cats. Clin Sci 61:169s–172s.
10 Angell-James JE, George MJ (1978) Carotid sinus baroreceptor control of blood pressure and vascular resistance in experimental cardiovascular disease and hypertension. IRCS Med Sci 6:160.
11 Mancia G, Ferrari A, Gregorini L, Zauchetti A (1979) Clonidine and carotid baroreflex in essential hypertension. Hypertension 1:362–370.
12 Korner PI (1981) Central nervous control of autonomic cardiovascular function. Handbook of physiology. The cardiovascular system I. Am Physiol Soc Chap 20: 691–739 (Washington, DC).

13 Mancia G, Parati G, Pomidossi G, Grassi G, Buccino N, Ferrari A, Gregorini L, Rupoli L, Zauchetti A (1982) Modification of arterial baroreflexes by captopril in essential hypertension. Am J Cardiol 49:1415–1419.

14 Mancia G, Ferrari A, Gregorini L, Ferrari MC, Bianchini C, Teizoli L, Leoretti G, Zauchetti A (1980) Effects of prazosin on autonomic control of circulation in essential hypertension. Hypertension 2:700–707

15 Mancia G (1983) Blood pressure variability at normal and high blood pressure. Chest 83:317S–320S.

16 Ferrari A, Gregorini L, Ferrari MC, Preti L, Mancia G (1981) Digitalis and baroreceptor reflexes in man. Circulation 63:279–285.

17 Ferrari A, Bonazzi O, Gregorini L, Gardinini M, Perondi R, Mancia G (1983) Modification of the baroreceptor control of atrio-ventricular conduction induced by digitalis in man. Cardiovascular Res 17:633–641.

Address for correspondence:
Professor G. Mancia
Istituto di Clinica Medica IV dell' Universita di Milano
Via F. Sforza, 35
20122 Milano
Italy

Discussion

HAYDUK:
Did you study the effects of digitalis in patients with cardiac insufficiency or in normal subjects?

MANCIA:
We studied normal subjects – mainly because patients with cardiac insufficiency would have had changes in stroke volume after treatment. It would then have been difficult to quantify the mechanical action of the baroreflexes.

KOBINGER:
We know from our own experiments on the baroreceptor reflex, that both major components of the autonomic nervous system are involved, resulting in a decrease in sympathetic activity and an increase in vagal activity. You measure the heart rate response, however, which is much more influenced by the vagus.

MANCIA:
This is exactly my point. Clonidine may enhance the baroreceptor vagal heart rate moderation. The blood pressure response which is dependent on sympathetic activity, was not enhanced. The last meeting on baroreceptors and hypertension terminated with the plea that we should stop talking about the baroreflex when we only measure the vagal component of the reflex because the two things may behave in a totally different fashion and may be affected in a different way.
I think this is also true in diabetic patients, for example, where the vagus is affected at a much earlier stage than the vasoconstrictor fibres.

PEART:
When you use peripheral resistance in discussing the action of drugs, do you think you have to take account of changes in muscle flow which might be substantially affected by what you are doing? I noticed that in your earlier studies peripheral resistance was calculated from cardiac output and blood pressure.

MANCIA:
I am afraid that we do not know where or to what extent the changes in muscle flow occur.

PEART:
Drugs which affect central sympathetic outflow lower peripheral resistance, and change blood pressure. I was wondering whether you had to take account, in your exercise studies, of the fact that there may be vast changes in muscle flow which are affected by the drugs.

MANCIA:
Yes, but I assume, although I am not sure, that vasodilation is the same before and after treatment because we keep the exercise the same. I would agree, however, that the determination of total peripheral resistance is a bad, indirect measurement but we use it in the absence of a superior measure.

Vascular autonomy and its relation to the action of antihypertensive drugs

J. G. Collier

Introduction

Raised peripheral resistance is a standard finding in patients with arterial hypertension and would account for the level of pressure at least in the chronic state. The mechanism for the increase in resistance remains obscure. Most theories have assumed that the vessels are constricted in response to disordered outside influences. Suggestions have included increased concentrations of the circulating constrictor substances adrenaline, noradrenaline, angiotensin II or the more recently described Na^+-K^+-ATPase inhibitor (de Wardener & MacGregor 1982). Alternatively increased levels of sympathetic nerve activity may be responsible, either because of some altered central mechanism, or because of altered peripheral control of mediator release (Brown & Macquin 1981). Some theories have considered that the abnormality may lie in the smooth muscle itself, and one popular hypothesis proposes that, at least in the chronic state, hypertension is maintained simply as a result of the physical bulk of the smooth muscle (Folkow 1978). Another hypothesis suggests that the smooth muscle has some specific abnormality of calcium handling (Robinson et al. 1982).

The possibility that there might be some imbalance in local mediator function has not been seriously considered. It has, however, become increasingly clear that blood vessels have, within their walls, a most intricate and subtle capacity to synthesize and metabolize vasoactive mediators that can directly constrict or dilate smooth muscle or act indirectly by modifying the function of nerve endings (Westfall 1977). The role of these local mediators has been recognized in the control of vessel tone in the inflammatory process (Williams & Peck 1977) and in the 'autoregulation' of blood flow through tissues (Sparks & Belloni 1978). In most circumstances such control can dominate systemic influence. As this potency is available under other circumstances it is perhaps naive to assume that in systemic disease peripheral vessels should necessarily be 'slave' to central or circulating mechanisms. In this article I will discuss the potential for vascular autonomy and relate it to some current ideas about the processes involved in the development of hypertension and to the action of certain antihypertensive drugs.

The renin-angiotensin system

Early work on the renin-angiotensin system suggested that raised circulating levels of angiotensin II (AII) might account for the increase in blood pressure at least in some patients. The predominant site for the production of this 'hypertensive' AII was thought to be the lungs. It was known that the lungs have an almost unlimited capacity to convert angiotensin I (AI) to AII (Biron et al. 1969). Therefore, assuming the provision of

51

sufficient levels of angiotensinogen (the precursor of AI), the rate-limiting factor in the system would be the concentration of circulating renin (measured in terms of plasma renin activity, PRA) delivered to the circulation by the juxta-glomerular apparatus (JGA) of the kidney. The concept of a dominant set of circulating controls began to be questioned with the observation in man, using local intraarterial and intravenous infusions of angiotensin I and II and the converting enzyme inhibitor SQ 20881, that the peripheral blood vessels had the capacity to convert AI to AII (Collier & Robinson 1974) and that this matched the conversion that occurred in the circulation as a whole when these drugs were given systemically (Collier et al. 1973). Furthermore these vessels, unlike the lungs were capable of inactivating AII (Vane 1969) which gave them enhanced control of the amount of mediator reaching and acting upon their own smooth muscle.

By means of cell cultures (Johnson 1980) and immunocytochemical and immunofluorescence techniques (Ryan & Ryan 1977) it has been shown that the capacity to convert AI into AII in vascular endothelial cells. This capacity varies between tissues, and appears to be greater in hypertensive than normotensive vasculature (Rosenthal et al. 1983).

The ability to convert inactive AI into the constrictor AII does not give the vessel autonomy unless it can also control the provision of AI and there is now good evidence to suggest that such local provision is feasible. Active renin has been detected in the walls of both arteries and veins (Dengler 1956; Gould et al. 1964; Assad & Antonaccio 1982) although it is still not clear whether it reaches the vessel from the plasma or is synthesized *de novo*. There is evidence to suggest that vessels can bind circulating renin and that the bound renin can remain active in the vessel for hours or days after the plasma renin has been removed (Assad & Antonaccio 1982). Arteries are more avid binders than veins and there is possibly more renin binding in vessels of hypertensive animals than in those that are normotensive (Basso et al. 1977; Assad & Antonaccio 1982). Such pharmacokinetics would effectively allow the vessel to act independently of circulating plasma renin. Indeed, several studies indicate that vascular renin activity may be raised when the renin level in the blood is low (Thurston & Swales 1977; Garst et al 1979; Assad & Antonaccio 1982). Moreover, in such circumstances blood pressure tends to correlate more closely with the renin in the vascular wall than with circulating renin levels (Garst et al. 1979; Assad & Antonaccio 1982).

Binding of circulating renin may not, however, be the sole means by which blood vessels obtain their supplies. The JGA can no longer be assumed to contain the only cells that can synthesize renin. Renin synthesis has now been shown to occur in brain tissue, in cultured chorionic (not amniotic) cells (Acker et al. 1982), and in the submaxillary gland, and of most relevance by cultured cells derived from the media of dog aorta (Haber 1980). If medial cells do synthesize renin, then the blood vessels have a second, more independent, way of determining their own AII levels.

Local vascular synthesis of renin might account for some important, but apparently paradoxical, observations. Firstly, at an epidemiological level, it seems that plasma renin is inversely proportional both to age and to blood pressure (certainly in white males and possibly in white females) (Meade et al. 1983). It is difficult to correlate this observation with the hypothesis that plasma renin has a direct role in controlling blood pressure in hypertensives and normotensives alike (MacGregor et al. 1979). This hypothesis is at least partially based on the effect of converting enzyme inhibition using captopril. Perhaps in some patients with low plasma renin the effect of the inhibitors is secondary to that of interference with vascular renin. Secondly and at a specifically clinical level, angiotensin converting enzyme inhibitors lower blood pressure in salt-depleted anephric patients, in whom there can be no levels of renal-derived renin (Man in't Veld et al. 1980). It is of interest that the hypotensive picture in these patients shifts from being predominantly that expected by arteriolar dilation to that suggesting venodilation. There is evidence that veins can harbour renin. Perhaps it is an unveiling of the renin in the vessel walls that is being observed in these patients.

Vascular renin, like renal renin, can be influenced by external agents, but the changes induced at the two renin sites are not similar. Whereas hydralazine and diuretics reduce vascular renin activity (Barrett et al 1978), they tend to increase plasma renin activity.

Although there is evidence that vessels contain renin, angiotensin converting enzyme, and enzymes capable of terminating the effect of formed AII, the vessels still depend on the circulation to provide supplies of angiotensinogen which is synthesized in the liver. This facultative provision should not be underestimated as the level of circulating angiotensinogen may be closely correlated with blood pressure (Gordon 1983). Such a correlation has been elegantly demonstrated in pregnant women where the level of the high molecular weight fraction of angiotensinogen closely followed blood pressure at a time when there was no significant change in plasma renin activity (Tewkesbury & Dart 1982). No drugs are yet available which selectively reduce angiotensinogen levels. It is interesting, however, that angiotensinogen levels rise in renal failure, and fall in hepatic failure, conditions associated with hypertension and hypotension respectively.

Arachidonic acid metabolism

It now seems likely that vessel walls have the full complement of enzymes needed to provide the complete arachidonic acid cascade. Of the 20 or more arachidonic acid derivatives that have been identified, three are of particular importance when considering the local control of blood vessel tone. The most potent dilator of this group of substances is prostacyclin (PGI_2) (Moncada et al. 1977). This is produced by the enzyme PGI_2 synthase which occurs in greatest abundance in endothelial cells, with smaller amounts in the media and adventitia (Herman et al. 1977). The substrates for PGI_2 synthase are the unstable peroxides PGG_2 and PGH_2 which are present locally and provided both by circulating platelets as they adhere to the endothelium and by local production in the vessel wall (Gryglewski et al. 1976). Any increase in the levels of the endoperoxides will increase PGI_2 synthesis; conversely when they diminish, PGI_2 levels fall. The vascular wall also contains the cyclo-oxygenase enzyme which is concerned with the production of the endoperoxides from arachidonic acid.

A second important arachidonic acid metabolite is thromboxane A_2, (TXA_2). Unlike PGI_2 this is a potent vasoconstrictor. It is produced from prostaglandin endoperoxides by the enzyme thromboxane synthase which is found predominantly in the adventitia and media. Little is present in the endothelium (Neri Serneri 1983). This site of synthesis gives easy access to the smooth muscle, but possibly makes TXA_2 less amenable to the effect of circulatory substances.

With the discovery of PGI_2 there was, as with renin, a desire to classify it as a 'circulating' hormone (Moncada et al. 1978). Early studies suggested that in man the main source of circulating PGI_2 was active secretion from the lungs (Hensby et al. 1979). It was reported that PGI_2 in blood or urine (measured in terms of the stable metabolite 6 oxo $F_{I\alpha}$) was lower in animals or patients with hypertension (Grose et al. 1980; Pace-Asciak & Carrara 1978). Thus a new candidate for the central control of vascular activity was suggested. However, with improved techniques and less enthusiasm, evidence now suggests that PGI_2 is probably not a circulating mediator of clinical importance since the blood levels being detected are too low to have any physiological effect (Fitzgerald et al. 1981). TXA_2, which is measured in terms of its more stable metabolite Thromboxane B_2, has also been reported to occur in the circulation, but as for PGI_2 levels detected in blood or urine, is probably best considered to be the result of an overflow from the vasculature and need not bear any direct relevance to local vascular levels and effects.

It is impossible to define the separate roles of these two prostaglandins *in vivo* since it is always possible that any effect detected clinically will be the sum of their opposing actions. Attempts have been made to look at their ratios in blood (Hornych et al. 1983) but such an approach, although attractive in that the results support the role of these arachidonic acid metabolites in the development of hypertension, suffers the same limitations as measureing the blood levels of the mediators singly.

An obvious approach to the assessment of the role of these cyclo-oxygenase-derived mediators, is to study the effects of sythesis inhibition. This is easily achieved by giving aspirin or other non-steroidal anti-inflammatory drugs (NSAIDs). Unfortunately, this approach is complicated by the presence of a third set of arachidonic acid derivatives, the leukotrienes. These are the component parts of the old SRSA which can now be identified individually. Recently the potent constrictor leukotriene B_4 (LTB_4) has been shown to be synthesized in vessel walls (Piper et al. 1983) and like the constrictor TXA_2 is found mainly in the adventitia and media. Although LTB_4 is synthesized from arachidonic acid it is different from PGI_2 and TXA_2 in that the enzyme responsible for producing the LTB_4 precursor is a lipoxygenase. This reaction is not blocked by NSAIDs; its synthesis might even be enhanced by them since they direct arachidonic acid to the LTB_4 pathway.

Faced with the difficulties of interpreting blood levels, and despite the selective nature of synthesis blockers available for use in man, indications of the functional significance of these mediators in vascular control has had to come from studies in which synthesis has been blocked by NSAIDs. The results of studies in which cyclo-oxygenase has been blocked suggest roles for endogenous vascular prostaglandins in the control of resting renal blood flow (Donker et al. 1976), in the vasodilatation associated with exercise (Kilbom & Wennmalm 1976) and ischaemia (Kilbom & Wennmalm 1976; Busse et al. 1983) and in the dilatation associated with the inflammatory process (Williams & Peck 1977). Their role in the control of blood pressure is less clear. Using a double blind protocol in normotensive volunteers, the intravenous infusion of indomethacin was found to cause a rise in arterial pressure which started within 3 minutes of beginning the infusion, persisted for the 10 minutes of the infusion, and gradually waned after the infusion was stopped (Wennmalm 1978). A similar rise in pressure is seen after intravenous indomethacin is given to animals (Collier, Personal observation). Cyclo-oxygenase inhibition not only prevents the synthesis of prostaglandins in blood vessel walls but also acts on the kidney to reduce renin release and cause salt and water retention (Lopez-Overojo et al. 1978). Clearly these renal effects would have secondary effects on blood pressure, although after acute administration a rapid rise in pressure could only be due to interference with the prostaglandins; the effects of salt and water retention would take too long to develop. Further support for the hypothesis that inhibition of prostaglandins is indeed the mechanism by which blood pressure is raised comes from two studies in which indomethacin was given to hypertensive patients over several weeks (Lopez-Overojo et al. 1978; Watkins et al. 1980). In both studies indomethacin had no effect alone, but in the presence of diuretics, which tend to reduce salt and water retention, it caused blood pressure to rise. Not all studies have detected rises in blood pressure after indomethacin or aspirin but in the face of the multitude of effects resulting from the administration of NSAIDs it is perhaps more surprising that positive responses have been reported at all.

Furchgott factor

The effects of certain vasoactive substances, notably acetycholine, are intimately related to the presence of vascular endothelial cells for, in their presence, acetylcholine is a potent dilator, in their absence, a constrictor (Furchgott 1981). The dilatation is mediated by a secondary substance released by the endothelial cells and carried to the smooth muscle. This substance, which has yet to be identified is not a prostaglandin, SRSA, or bradykinin. Evidence for its release has been found in numerous tissues from different species and in addition to mediating responses to acetylcholine, it contributes to the responses to bradykinin and adenosine. Part of the dilator effect of hydralazine is secondary to production of this endothelial factor, even though some residual dilatation occurs in the absence of such cells (Spokas et al. 1983). The endothelial cells can also act to modify the response to constrictors; their removal can potentiate the constrictor effect of noradrenaline (Verrecchia et al. 1983; Cocks & Angus 1983) and 5-HT (Cohen et al. 1983; Cocks & Angus 1983). Animal studies suggest that release of the Furchgott factor can be caused by stimulation of endothelial α_2 or 5-HT receptors (Cocks & Angus 1983); such a mechanism has obvious relevance to the hypotensive effect of the α_2-agonist clonidine. It might be that in hypertensives Furchgott factor production (or activity) is reduced. This would account for the increased sensitivity of hypertensive patients to infusions of noradrenaline (Doyle et al. 1959; Sivertsson 1970) and would allow increased apparent sympathetic activity wihout detectable changes in noradrenaline release. Reduction in the factor might also be the cause of the reduced sensitivity to hydralazine seen in some hypertensive patients after a few weeks therapy (Robinson et al. 1980).

Endothelial cells are fragile, easily removed by rubbing with a balloon catheter, and take up to 70 days to regenerate (Elder et al. 1981). They have diverse biochemical activity which, until recently, has been ignored. This may be because they have been unwittingly removed or damaged in many of the *in vitro* studies of vascular behaviour. Minor impairment in their function might contribute to changes in vessel tone.

Conclusion

There is abundant evidence that blood vessels have in their walls the wherewithal to synthesize and metabolize vasoactive mediators and to modify the response to drugs. Many mediators have potent direct effects on smooth muscle, some also interfere with

55

the release of mediators from nerve endings. It is likely that many influence other synthetic pathways. It is difficult to believe that such mediators, strategically placed at the site of smooth muscle contraction, would not influence vascular tone both in normal subjects and in those with hypertension. The capacity of drugs to selectively modify the processes involved in these pathways must certainly enhance understanding and may lead to advances in therapeutics.

References

1 Acker GM, Galen FX, Devaux C, Foote S, Papernik E, Pesty A, Menard J, Corval P (1982) Human chorionic cells in primary culture: a model for renin biosynthesis. J Clin Endocrinol Metab 55:902–909.
2 Asaad MM, Antonaccio MJ (1982) Vascular wall renin in spontaneously hyptertensive rats. Hypertension 4:487–493.
3 Barrett JD, Eggena P, Sambhi MP (1978) Partial characterisation of aortic renin in the spontaneously hypertensive rat and its interrelationship with plasma renin, blood pressure and sodium balance. Clin Sci Molec Med 55:261–270.
4 Basso N, Lurnjek M, Tagnini AC (1977) Vascular renin-like activity and blood pressure. Mayo Clin Proc 52:437–441.
5 Biron P, Campeau L, David P (1969) Fate of angiotensin I and II in the human pulmonary circulation. Am J Cardiol 24:544–547.
6 Brown MJ, Macquin I (1981) Is adrenaline the cause of essential hypertension? Lancet ii:1079–1082.
7 Busse R, Pohl U, Holtz J, Bassenge E (1983) Hypoxic dilation of coronary arteries in vitro mediated by endothelium. Blood Vessels 20:188.
8 Cocks TM, Angus JA (1983) Endothelium-dependent relaxation of coronary arteries by noradrenaline and serotonin. Nature 305:627–630.
9 Cohen RA, Shepherd JT, Vanhoutte PM (1983) Inhibitory role of endothelium in response of isolated canine coronary arteries to platelets. Blood Vessels 20:188–189.
10 Collier JG, Robinson BF (1974) Comparison of effects of locally infused angiotensin I and II on hand veins and forearm arteries in man: evidence for converting enzyme activity in limb vessels. Clin Sci Molec Med 47:189–192.
11 Collier JG, Robinson BF, Vane JR (1973) Reduction of pressor effects of angiotensin I in man by synthetic nonapeptide (B.P.P.$_{9a}$ or SQ 20,881) which inhibits converting enzyme. Lancet i:72–79.
12 Dengler H (1956) Über einen reinartigen Wirkstoff in Arterienextrakten. Naunyn-Schmiedenbergs Arch Exp Pathol Pharmakol 227:481–487.
13 de Wardener HE, MacGregor GA (1982) The natriuretic hormone and essential hypertension. Lancet i:1450–1454.
14 Donker AJM, Arisz L, Brentjens JRH, van der Hem GK, Hollemans HJG (1976) The effect of indomethacin on kidney function and plasma renin activity in man. Nephron 17:288–296.
15 Doyle AE, Fraser JRE, Marshall RJ (1959) Reactivity of forearm vessels to vasoconstrictor substances in hypertensive and normotensive subjects. Clin Sci 18:441–454.
16 Eldor A, Falcone DJ, Hajjar DP, Minnick CR, Weksler BB (1981) Recovery of prostacyclin production by de-endothelialised rabbit aorta. Critical role of neo-intimal smooth muscle cells. J Clin Invest 67:735–741.
17 FitzGerald GA, Brash AR, Falardeau P, Oates JA (1981) Estimated rate of prostacyclin secretion into the circulation of normal man. J Clin Invest 68:1271–1276.
18 Folkow B (1978) Cardiovascular structural adaptation; its role in the initiation and maintenance of primary hypertension. Clin Sci Mol Med 55 (Suppl 4):3s–22s.
19 Furchgott RF (1981) The requirement for endothelial cells in the relaxation of arteries by acetylcholine and some other vasodilators. TIPS July:173–176.
20 Garst JB, Koletsky S, Wisenbaugh PE, Hadady M, Mathews D (1979) Arterial wall renin and renal venous renin in the hypertensive rat. Clin Sci Mol Med 56:41–46.
21 Gordon DB (1983) The role of renin substrate in hypertension. Hypertension 5:353–362.

22 Gould AB, Skeggs LT, Kahn JR (1964) The presence of renin activity in blood vessel walls. J Exp Med 119:389–399.

23 Grose JH, Lebel M, Gbeassor FM (1980) Diminished urinary prostacyclin metabolite in essential hypertension. Clin Sci (Suppl 6) 59:121s–123s.

24 Gryglewski RJ, Bunting S, Moncade S, Flower RJ, Vane JR (1976) Arterial walls are protected against deposition of platelet thrombi by a substance (prostaglandin X) which they make from prostaglandin endoperoxides. Prostaglandins 12:685–713.

25 Haber E (1980) Specific inhibitors of renin. Clin Sci (Suppl 6) 59:7s–19s.

26 Hensby CN, Barnes PJ, Dollery CT, Dargie H (1979) Production of 6 oxo $PGF_{1\alpha}$ by human lung in vivo. Lancet ii:1162–1163.

27 Herman AG, Moncada S, Vane JR (1977) Formation of prostacyclin (PGI_2) by different layers of the arterial wall. Arch Int Pharmacodyn 227:162–163.

28 Hornych A, Safar M, Levenson J, Simon A, London G, Bariety J (1983) Proceedings of the Hypertension Congress, Milan. Abstract 190.

29 Johnson AR (1980) Human pulmonary endothelial cells in culture: activities of cells from arteries and cells from veins. J Clin Invest 65:841–850.

30 Kilbom Å, Wennmalm A (1976) Endogenous prostaglandins as local regulators of blood flow in man: effect of indomethacin on reactive and functional hyperaemia. J Physiol 257:109–121.

31 Lopez-Overojo JA, Weber MA, Drayer JIM, Sealey JE, Laragh JH (1978) Effect of indomethacin alone and during diuretic or β-adrenoceptor blockade therapy on blood pressure and the renin system in essential hypertension. Clin Sci Molec Med 55 (Suppl 4):203s–205s.

32 MacGregor GA, Markandu ND, Roulston JE (1979). Does the renin-angiotensin system maintain blood pressure in both hypertensive and normotensive subjects? A comparison of propranolol, saralasin and captopril. Clin Sci 57:145–148.

33 Man in't Veld AJ, Schicht IM, Derkx FHM, De Bruyn JHB, Schalekamp MADH (1980) Effects of angiotensin converting enzyme inhibitor (captopril) on blood pressure in anephric subjects. Br Med J 280:288–290.

34 Meade TW, Imeson JD, Gordon D, Peart WS (1983) The epidemiology of plasma renin. Clin Sci 64:273–280.

35 Moncada S, Higgs EA, Evans JR (1977) Human arterial and venous tissues generate prostacyclin (prostaglandin X), a potent inhibitor of platelet aggregation. Lancet i:18–20.

36 Moncada S, Korbut R, Bunting S, Vane JR (1978) Prostacyclin is a circulating hormone. Nature 273:767–768.

37 Neri Serneri GG, Abbate R, Gensini GF, Panetta A, Casolo GC, Carini M (1983) TXA_2 production by human arteries and veins. Prostaglandins 25:754–766.

38 Pace-Asciak CR, Carrara MC (1978) Evidence suggesting a systemic antihypertensive role for PGI_2. Prostaglandins 15:704.

39 Piper PJ, Letts LG, Galton SA (1983) Generation of a leukotriene-like substance from porcine vascular and other tissues. Prostaglandins 25:591–599.

40 Robinson BF, Collier JG, Dobbs RJ (1980) Acquired tolerance to dilator action of hydralazine during oral administration. Br J Clin Pharmacol 9:407–412.

41 Robinson BF, Dobbs RJ, Bayley S (1982) Response of forearm resistance vessels to verapamil and sodium nitroprusside in normotensive and hypertensive men: evidence for a functional abnormality in primary hypertension. Clin Sci 63:33–42.

42 Ryan JW, Ryan US (1977) Pulmonary endothelial cells. Fed Proc 36:2683–2691.

43 Sivertsson R (1970) The haemodynamic importance of structural vascular changes in essential hypertension. Acta Physiol Scand 343:whole issue.

44 Sparks HV, Belloni FL (1978) The peripheral circulation: local regulation. Ann Rev Physiol 40:67–92.

45 Spokas EG, Folco G, Quilley J, Chander P, McGiff JC (1983) Endothelial mechanism in the vascular action of hydralazine. Hypertension 5:I 107–111.

46 Tewksbury DA, Dart RA (1982) High molecular weight angiotensinogen levels in hypertensive pregnant women. Hypertension 4:729–734.

47 Thurston H, Swales JD (1977) Blood pressure response of nephrectomised hypertensive rats to converting enzyme inhibition: evidence for persistent vascular renin activity. Clin Sci Molec Med 52:299–304.

57

48 Vane JR (1969) The release and fate of vasoactive hormones in the circulation. Br J Pharmac 35:209–242.
49 Verrechia C, Sercombe R, Seylaz J (1983) Endothelium removal enhances norepinephrine vasoconstriction. Blood Vessels 20:210.
50 Watkins J, Carl Abbott EC, Hensby CN, Webster J, Dollery CT (1980) Attenuation of hypotensive effect of propranolol and thiazide diuretics by indomethacin. Br Med J 281:702–705.
51 Wennmalm A (1978) Influence of indomethacin on the systemic and pulmonary vascular resistance in man. Clin Sci Molec Med 54:141–145.
52 Westfall TC (1977) Local regulation of adrenergic neurotransmission. Physiol Rev 57:659–727.
53 Williams TJ, Peck MJ (1977) Role of prostaglandin-mediated vasodilatation in inflammation. Nature 270:530–532.

Correspondence:
Dr. J. G. Collier
Department of Pharmacology
St George's Hospital Medical School
London SW17 ORE
U.K.

Discussion

MATHIAS:
I am fascinated by your description of the Furchgott Factor. What is the half life of this factor? The reason I ask is that if a prolonged infusion of noradrenaline is given and then suddenly stopped, the blood pressure falls precipitously, previous workers including Professor Peart, have wondered about the possible existence of a circulating vasodilator substance. This may also partly explain the marked fall in blood pressure in phaeochromocytoma patients immediately after tumour removal, especially if the half-life of such a factor is longer than that of noradrenaline.

COLLIER:
I think that nobody knows. We know of such a factor only because removal of the endothelial cells reverses acetylcholine or bradykinin or adenosine responses. Equally, if you put two tissues together the substance apparently passes between one tissue and the other and therefore it is supposed to be transmissible. I do not know whether this happens in man but noradrenaline enhancement has been shown in animals.

PEART:
Certainly the blood pressure fall attended by marked flushing does raise that possibility: a very marked flush is seen in man as you probably know. Mowbray and I had thought that there was a vasodilator produced, to explain why, when you infused, the blood pressure fell fairly steadily and if you increased the dose of noradrenaline it was difficult to maintain a fixed level of blood pressure.
We thought that we had demonstrated such an effect on isolated muscle in the dog, but this obviously takes it a lot further.

COLLIER:
You can only assume a dilator effect because removal of the endothelial cells causes a greater constrictor response than normal but these studies were in animals and clearly man should be studied next.

TUCK:
When you talk about the steroid effect on arachidonic acid and blood pressure do you mean glucocorticoids?

COLLIER:
Yes.

TUCK:
Is this a rapid effect on blood pressure?

COLLIER:
The observation is that if you give corticosteroids, the pressure goes up – that is a well-recognized effect – and it takes at least 4–6 hours for that effect to bew seen because there is an intermediary step when the steroids produce a second substance called macrocortin. It could be that the rise in pressure is related to this but there are alternatives such as salt and water retention.

General discussion

WEBER:

Have there been any studies to suggest that long-term treatment with antihypertensive agents such as clonidine will bring about some permanent change in baroreflexes? Has there been an opportunity to see if the intrinsic nature of the hypertension has been altered by the treatment?

GUTHRIE:

This touches on some of the differences between our studies and those of others. Our patients were studied after one month of treatment; other studies, such as Dr Mancia's, were after an intravenous injection and I think that this is important. The bulk of the evidence suggests that in many patients with hypertension, resetting of the baroreflex by treatment may be the result of lowering the blood pressure alone. That would be a criticism of our studies. We undertook the prazosin studies as the control, assuming that prazosin had only a peripheral action and on finding that the baroreflex was unaffected we assumed that they were an appropriate control to the studies with sustained clonidine treatment. However, other studies, but without suitable controls with reduced blood pressure over the long term, found a sustained reduction and alteration of baroreflex. We have not, however, studied the baroreflex longer than one month following treatment. Whether this reduction is maintained beyond that point we just do not know.

MANCIA:

I think that this is an important point. Our studies with clonidine were acute studies. The studies with other drugs were chronic studies and by chronic I mean two weeks' treatment and no more. I think that in Dr Guthrie's study, the people were on treatment for somewhat longer. It is very important because the mechanisms of baroreflex control, as studied in animals, are very complex. It may be that changes in the viscoelastic properties of the vessel wall may cause an anatomical resetting.

KOBINGER:

In animals the resetting of the baroreceptors appears to be due to stimulation of medullary alpha adrenoceptors and I assume that the effect lasts as long as the drug is acting on the central nervous system.

WEBER:

A number of speakers this morning – Dr Collier, Dr Mathias, Professor Peart – talked about the interaction between the renin-angiotensin system and the catecholamines or the sympathetic nervous system. What is the latest thinking on how this interaction works? Is it that the angiotensin is in some way preventing re-uptake of noradrenaline preynaptically or is it preventing its metabolism postsynaptically or possibly enhancing its potency at the receptor? Do we have any up-to-date ideas on how that is working?

MATHIAS:

There is a large amount of *in vitro* data which indicates that in the periphery angiotensin II can enhance release of noradrenaline, can decrease its clearance and uptake and thus result in a greater vascular response. I am not aware of studies which have extended these observations in man but perhaps Dr Collier might be able to comment.

COLLIER:

That seems to be the case. The other thing is that angiotensin acts on the brain and causes the release of catecholamines peripherally, particularly in some vessels such as those in the hand.

MATHIAS:

In the central nervous system, there is a considerable amount of work on sites of action of angiotensin II and its effects on the sympathetic nervous system not only directly but via the interaction of various other peptides such as the opioids. Studies in man are limited but further studies, from our own group and elsewhere, are now addressing these potentially important effects.

60

MANCIA:

I would like to ask for Dr Mathias' view on what really happens to the spinal cord mechanisms after transection at the cervical level? Do they regain their activity tonically and phasically? Tonically, it seems that they do not. Can we interpret these huge responses as an index of the ability of the sympathetic neurons of the intermediolateral column to be excited by afferent fibres or is it only a peripheral phenomenon?

MATHIAS:

Initially, and this is where the responses differ from those of animals, there is a state of spinal shock – we have looked at this in some detail previously – and, we cannot activate the sympathetic nervous system at a spinal level. This lasts for about 4–6 weeks, on average, before the second or chronic phase during which there is no doubt that different afferent stimuli induce marked effects. The studies I described involved activating the urinary bladder; stimulating different viscera, or inducing muscle spasms certainly produce spinal reflex activity. There is no doubt that it is a spinal reflex on the basis of physiological and pharmacological studies. Different drugs block different sites. Lignocaine, for instance, in the urinary bladder blocks the afferents and prevents hypertension. So also do ganglion blocking agents. This very clearly indicates the involvement of spinal sympathetic reflexes. The sympathetic nerve terminals appear to function adequately as far as we can tell: histochemical studies indicate that they are no different from those in normal man. So I think that we are observing the responses to afferent stimuli which are much greater than in normal man. To what extent these reflexes influence blood pressure regulation either in normal subjects or hypertensives remains to be determined.

PEART:

Could I tempt Collier to comment on Bayliss who was perhaps the first to go into the question of local regulation? What he said has not really been challenged or modified much over the years. Bayliss pointed out that when you lower the perfusing pressure through a vessel, it dilates and when you raise the pressure, it constricts: the phenomenon of local autoregulation independent of nerves. How would you like to fit that into your hypothesis?

COLLIER:

We do not know what this endothelial tissue does in response to stretch. The whole area of local control even in terms of post-ischaemic hyperaemia has only been nibbled at. We can add antihistamines but it's still there and we can add aspirin but it's still there. We are left with an enormous amount of postischaemic hyperaemia which is not explained. Even if you add calcium blockers, it changes, but it's still there. So there is still plenty of work to be done.

PEART:

What interests me is that you have cells responding to a change of pressure. In physiological terms, we are not used to biochemical change being brought about by stretch. What is it about stretch which would bring about a biochemical change, do you think?

COLLIER:

If you touch, tickle or stretch a lung it releases an enormous amount of prostaglandins – that is physical – it was done originally by Priscilla Piper and one wondered if it was her particular way of inflating the lungs, but other people have repeated it.

Therapeutic consequences

Chairman: S. S. Franklin

Therapeutic decisions in mild hypertension: an introductory overview

S. S. Franklin

This introductory overview of mild hypertension will deal with the related issues of whom to treat and how to treat. Intervention trials have not so far given clear guidelines for the effective treatment of mild hypertension. Perhaps these studies have been flawed by the nature of their design; they have tried to achieve the combined goal of statistical validity and wide applicability in diverse groups of hypertensive patients. Moreover, the risk factor concept involves a statement of group probability so that some patients at low risk develop cardiovascular complications and others at high risk do not.

The level varies at which it is recommended to treat mild hypertension; 90 mm Hg diastolic blood pressure and above was recommended in the United States HDFP intervention study (1979 a and b; 1982), 95 mm Hg diastolic blood pressure and above in the Australian Thereapeutic Trial (1980) and 100 mm Hg diastolic or higher in the Oslo trial (Helgeland 1980). Reviews of intervention trials have shown that the most convincing evidence of effective therapy is found in subjects over 50 years of age with a diastolic blood pressure of 100 mm Hg or more, in association with hypertensive target organ damage and other cardiovascular risk factors (Alderman and Madhavan 1981; Freis 1982; Peart 1981). In contrast, the Build and Blood Pressure Actuary Study of 1979 (Society of Actuaries and Association of Life Insurance Medical Directors of America 1980), suggested that in comparison with normotensive controls, freedom from hypertensive risk does not disappear after initiating therapy until blood pressure values of 127 mm Hg systolic and 83 mm Hg diastolic are reached. Thus, clear guidelines for therapeutic intervention in the patient with mild hypertension have not been established.

How can we improve decision-making in the treatment of mild hypertension? There are two approaches which show promise. First, there are now improved methods of blood pressure classification. The recent work of Perloff et al. (1983) with an automatic blood-pressure recording device has shown better correlation of ambulatory blood pressure with both fatal and non-fatal cardiovascular events, compared with casual 'office' blood pressure measurements. In 78% of patients ambulatory blood pressures were lower than casual office blood pressure, while in the remaining 22% the ambulatory blood pressure was the same or higher than office readings. Moreover, the study of Devereux et al. (1983) has shown a closer correlation of left ventricular hypertrophy with ambulatory blood pressure at work than with casual, home, or sleep blood pressure.

Decision-making can also be improved by using better methods of assessing the attributable risk of hypertension; this represents the risk of hypertension that is not directly confounded by other cardiovascular risk factors. Table 1 shows the natural history of blood pressure in placebo-treated, mildly hypertensive paitents in three intervention trials (The Australian Therapeutic Trial in Mild Hypertension 1980; Smith

Table 1. Natural history of placebo-treated mild hypertension.

Study	Number of patients	Duration of study (years)	Acceleration of hypertension (%)	
			Placebo group	Treated group
Veterans Administration Cooperative Study group on Antihypertensive Agents (1970)	170	3.9	12 Diastolic blood pressure ≧ 124 mm Hg	0.0
United States Public Health Trial (Smith 1977)	196	> 7	18 Diastolic blood pressure ≧ 130 mm Hg	0.5
The Australian Therapeutic Trial in Mild Hypertension (1980)	1706	3.8	12 Systolic blood pressure > 199 mm Hg or diastolic blood pressure > 190 mm Hg	0.3

1977; Veterans Administration Cooperative Study Group on Antihypertensive Agents 1970). Note that a significant worsening of hypertension, commonly associated with hypertensive retinopathy, occurs at the rate of approximately 3% per year in the placebo groups, whereas it is largely eliminated in patients receiving antihypertensive drugs. At the present time we are unable to predetermine which hypertensive patients are destined to develop accelerating hypertension. Perhaps the use of ambulatory monitoring of blood pressure will be useful in this context.

One of the earliest measured of hypertensive risk is the development of left-ventricular hypertrophy. Table 2 shows the influence of hypertension on left-ventricular hypertrophy in two intervention trials. In the United States Public Health Trial (Smith 1977), which lasted seven years, an additional 7.4% of the placebo control group developed left-ventricular hypertrophy as diagnosed by ECG, in comparison with the treatment group. Similarly, over the five years of the Hypertension Detection and Follow-up Program (Polk 1982) the community control group (referred care) showed an additional 4.5% of left-ventricular hypertrophy, in comparison with the intensely treated step-care group. Even more impressive was the percentage of regression of left-ventricular hypertrophy in patients receiving treatment for their hypertension, with step-care showing 60% and referred care 49%. Predictably, the less intensely treated referred care group showed 11% less regression of left-ventricular hypertrophy than did the step-care patient.

Recent studies have shown that the echocardiogram is far more sensitive than either chest radiograph or ECG for the diagnosis of left-ventricular hypertrophy (Savage et al. 1979). Using echocardiography, Laird and Fixler (1981) diagnosed left-ventricular hypertrophy in 16% of 50 young adolescents with mild hypertension (average blood pressure 134 mm Hg systolic and 91 mm Hg diastolic), though no cases were found in 50 matched normotensive control subjects. Thus, the echocardiogram may become an excellent tool in the diagnosis of early hypertensive risk.

Table 2. Influence of hypertension on left-ventricular hypertrophy (LVH)

Study	Diagnostic technique	Treatment group (end of study)	Control group (end of study)	Attributable risks
United States Public Health Trial (Smith 1977)	EGG	15.7% LVH	23.1% LVH	7.4% LVH per 7 years
Hypertension Detection and Follow-up Program Cooperative Study (1979 a and b; 1982)	ECG	4.1% LVH (SC) 60.3% regression of LVH (SC)	8.6% LVH (RC) 49.2% regression of LVH (RC)	4.5% LVH per 5 years 11.1% LVH regression per 5 year

SC = step care
RC = referred care

67

Finally, one important question remains unanswered: does hypertensive risk correlate with mild hypertension of long duration, or with the propensity for mild hypertension to rise to moderate and severe levels prior to the development of cardiovascular morbidity? Studies have not so far adequately addressed this important issue.

Decision-making in the treatment of mild hypertension has recently become more controversial. There are two basic questions which need to be answered. First, what is the success of nonpharmacological therapy, such as behavioural modification, weight reduction, or low-sodium diets, in the management of the hypertensive patient? To summarize briefly, behavioural modification has not yet been shown to be any more effective in lowering blood pressure than placebo controls (Shapiro 1980). In contrast, weight reduction and moderate low-sodium diets have been shown to lower blood pressure significantly more than in placebo controls (MacGregor et al. 1982; Reisin et al. 1978); however, neither the community response rate nor the rate of recidivism have yet been determined (Strunkard 1980). One must therefore conclude that weight reduction and low-sodium diets are useful forms of therapy during the initial period of blood pressure observation and classification, which can extend over many months. Beyond that point, if successful blood pressure control has not been achieved, one should consider these measures as adjuncts to drug treatment.

The second basic question concerns the side-effects of antihypertensive agents. Drug therapy may have undesirable risks which must be matched against their benefits. The ideal antihypertensive agent should lower blood pressure in a physiological manner, produce no increased risk of cardiovascular or non-cardiovascular disease, and produce no significant impairment in the quality of life. Recently, the use of diuretics as a first step in step-care therapy has come under attack, perhaps for the wrong reasons. The Multiple Risk Factor Intervention Trial (MRFIT) (1982), recently completed in the United States, has attributed a higher incidence of sudden death from myocardial infarction to the use of diuretic therapy. If this association is correct, and it should be noted that the MRFIT study is not statistically valid, it would appear to be due to the inappropriate use of very high doses of diuretic rather than to the inherent toxocity of the drugs. A more convincing reason for beginning therapy with other agents is that in certain subsets of hypertensive patients, they may be more effective and have fewer side-effects than diuretics. One must remember, however, that as many as 50% of mild-tomoderate hypertensives will require at least two drugs for optimal control of their hypertension; a diuretic may be a logical choice for one of these agents (Dolhery 1981).

The matching of patient profiles to a specific antihypertensive drug, rather than using empirical step-care therapy, appears to be gaining in popularity. Since the emphasis of this symposium is on the role of central alpha$_2$-agonists, particularly clonidine, in the treatment of hypertension, it is appropriate to examine the properties of this agent which may be relevant to specific clinical problems, as follows.

(1) Clonidine lowers blood pressure by activating alpha$_2$-adrenergic receptors in the cardiovascular control centre of the brain, resulting in suppression of sympathetic outflow to the cardiovascular system. Rapid onset of action is ensured by the small molecular size and high lipid solubility of clonidine, which allows the drug to enter the vasomotor centre rapidly via the area postrema without having to cross the blood-brain barrier (Davis et al. 1977) This property makes clonidine useful in treating symptomatic paroxysmal hypertension, as well as hypertensive emergencies (Anderson et al. 1981; Bravo et al. 1981).

(2) Since baroreceptor reflex function is not impaired, and may actually be enhanced by clonidine (Ebringer et al. 1970; Mancia et al. 1979), there are no increased orthostatic symptoms in the elderly or diabetic patient, who may already have some impairment of orthostatic reflex control.

(3) Any reduction in cardiac output after clonidine administration is secondary to vagally-induced decreased heart rate; there is no impairment of myocardial contractility, and therefore a normal response to exercise and no aggravation of congestive heart failure (Lambie and Schmitt 1974).

(4) Because suppression of sympathetic activity with clonidine results in a favourable shift of the arterial pressure – renal sodium excretion curve (Guyton et al. 1974; Itskovitz 1980), a long-term negative salt and water balance may occur, despite decreased renal perfusion pressures (Campese et al. 1980; Miller 1980). Thus, a rapid lowering of blood pressure secondary to altered sympathetic vascular tone may be reinforced by secondary natriuresis.

Thus, if a hyperactive central sympathetic nervous system plays a key role in initiating essential hypertension, down regulation of sympathetic activity with central alpha$_2$-agonists would appear to provide a physiological approach to therapy. Newer agents such as angiotensin-converting enzyme inhibitors and calcium antagonists lower blood pressure sufficiently, but the limited experience with these drugs precludes an adequate estimation of risk at this time.

Finally, the important problem of treatment compliance must be solved before successful community control of hypertension can be achieved. It should be remembered that proper selection of the dose and timing of administration may help to minimize undesirable side-effects and thereby enhance compliance.

Summary

Hypertension is not easily classified in terms of attributable cardiovascular risk. Previous approaches to the treatment of mild hypertension with drugs have resulted in errors of both omission and commission, and the subject remains controversial. Improved methods of determining hypertensive risk must be established; perhaps ambulatory blood pressure recording and echocardiogram screening for early left-ventricular hypertrophy will help to solve this problem. The conventional step-care approach must be re-evaluated. The risk/benefit ratio also deserves careful consideration in deciding which drug to use. Specific study of the hypertensive patient, with attention to changes in physiological responses, should be of value in drug selection.

References

1 Alderman MH, Madhavan MS (1981) Management of the hypertensive patient: a continuing dilemma. Hypertension 3:192–197.
2 Anderson RJ, Hart GH, Crumpler CP, Reed WG, Matthews CA (1981) Oral clonidine loading in hypertensive urgencies. JAMA 246:848–850.
3 Bravo EL, Tarazi RC, Fouad FM, Vidt DG, Gifford RW (1981) Clonidine-suppression test, a useful aid in the diagnosis of pheochromocytoma. N Engl J Med 305:623–626.

4 Campese VM, Romoff M, Telfer N, Weidman P, Massry SG (1980) Role of sympathetic nerve inhibition and body sodium-volume state in the antihypertensive action of clonidine in essential hypertension. Kidney Int 18:351–357.

5 Davis DS, Wing LMH, Reid JL, Neill E, Tippett P, Dollery CT (1977) Pharmacokinetics and concentration-effect relationships of intravenous and oral clonidine. Clin Pharmacol Ther 21:593–601.

6 Devereux RB, Pickering TG, Harshfielf GA (1983) Left ventricular hypertrophy in patients with hypertension: importance of blood pressure response to regularly recurring stress. Circulation 68:470–476.

7 Dollery CT (1981) Does it matter how blood pressure is reduced? Clin Sci 61:413s–420s.

8 Ebringer A, Dolye AE, Dawborn JK, Johnston CI, Mashford ML (1970) The use of clonidine in the treatment of hypertension. Med J Aust 1:523–530.

9 Freis ED (1982) Should mild hypertension be treated? N Engl J Med 307:306–309.

10 Guyton AC, Cowley Jr AW, Coleman TG et al. (1974) Hypertension: a disease of abnormal circulatory control. Chest 65:328–338.

11 Helgeland A (1980) Treatment of mild hypertension: a five-year controlled study. Am J Med 69:725–732.

12 Hypertension Detection and Follow-up Program Cooperative Study (1979a) Five-year findings of the hypertension detection and follow-up program. Reduction of mortality in persons with high blood pressure including mild hypertension. JAMA 242:2562–2571.

13 Hypertension Detection and Follow-up Program Cooperative Study (1979b) Five-year findings of the hypertension detection and follow-up program, II. Mortality by race – sex and age. JAMA 242:2572–2577.

14 Hypertension Detection and Follow-up Program Cooperative Study (1982) The effects of treatment on mortality in 'mild' hypertension. N Engl J Med 307:976–980.

15 Itskovitz D (1980) Renal effects of clonidine. J Cardiovasc Pharmacol 2 (Suppl 1):S47–S60.

16 Laird WP, Fixler DE (1981) Left-ventricular hypertrophy in adolescents with elevated blood pressure: assessment by chest roentgenography, electrocardiography, and echocardiography. Pediatrics 67:255–259.

17 Laubie M, Schmitt H (1974) Influence of autonomic blockade on the reduction in myocardial performance produced by clonidine. Eur J Pharmacol 25:56–60.

18 Mancia G, Ferrari A, Gregorini A, Zanchetti A (1979) Clonidine and carotid baroreflex in essential hypertension. Hypertension 1:362–370.

19 Miller M (1980) Clonidine-induced diuresis in the rat: evidence for a renal site of action. J Pharmacol Exp Ther 214:608–613.

20 Multiple Risk Factor Intervention Trial Research Group (1982) Multiple Risk factor intervention trial. JAMA 248:1465–1477.

21 MacGregor GA, Markandu ND, Best FE et al. (1982) Double-blind randomised crossover trial of moderate sodium restriction in essential hypertension. Lancet i:351–354.

22 Peart WS (1981) The problem of treatment in mild hypertension Clin Sci 61:403s–411s.

23 Perloff D, Sokolow M, Cowan R (1983) The prognostic value of ambulatory blood pressures. JAMA 249:2792–2798.

24 Polk B (1982) Effect of antihypertensive medication of left-ventricular hypertrophy. Am J Epidemiol 116:579.

25 Reisin E, Abel R, Modan M, Silverberg DS, Eliahou HE, Modan B (1978) Effect of weight loss without salt restriction on the reduction of blood pressure in overweight hypertensive patients. N Engl J Med 298:1–60.

26 Savage DD, Drayer JIM, Henry WL et al. (1979) Echocardiographic assessment of cardiac anatomy and function in hypertensive subjects. Circulation 59:623–632.

27 Shapiro AP (1980) Behaviour modification: can it control hypertension? J Cardiovasc Med 12:1075–1079.

28 Society of Actuaries and Association of Life Insurance Medical Directors of America (1980) Build and Blood Pressure Study 1979. Recording and Statistical Corp, USA.

29 Strunkard AJ (1980) Obesity and social environment: current status, future prospects. In: Bray GA (ed) Obesity in America: a conference. NIH Publication No. 80–359, May.

30 The Australian Therapeutic Trial in Mild Hypertension (1980) Lancet i:1261–1267.

31 Smith WF (1977) Treatment of Mild Hypertension: results of a ten-year intervention trial. Circ Res 40 (Suppl 1):98–105.
32 Veterans Administration Cooperative Study Group of Antihypertensive Agents (1970) Effects of treatment on morbidity in hypertension. II. Results in patients with diastolic blood pressure averaging 90 through 114 mm Hg. JAMA 213:1143–1152.

Correspondence:
Stanley S. Franklin, M. D.
Adjunct Professor of Medicine and Associate Director of Hypertension
University of California at Los Angeles, USA.

When to treat? Recent trials in mild hypertension. Epidemiological data and conclusions

K. Hayduk

Introduction

The aim of treatment of mild hypertension is to lower the incidence of cardiovascular events by reduction of blood pressure. This aim can be achieved (Australian Therapeutic Trial in Mild Hypertension 1980; HDFP Study 1979 a, b, 1982 a, b). Nevertheless the possible side-effects of antihypertensive treatment must be considered. The quality of life of the patients is important especially since mild hypertension on its own is a relatively weak risk factor for the individual patient despite its high incidence in the community.

When treating mild hypertension the degree of benefit also has to be taken into account. The method of demonstrating the effect of treatment has a significant influence on the apparent outcome. For example, in the HDFP study (1979 a, b, 1982 a, b), the cardiovascular mortality was reduced in stepped care patients (active group) *by* about 20% compared to referred care (control group). However, this refers to a reduction in mortality from 7.7 to 6.4%, that is *of* only 1.3% (the 'of or by' dilemma (Pickering 1983)).

Intervention trials

In earlier intervention trials (Berglund et al. 1978; Veterans' Administration Cooperative Study Group on Antihypertensive Agents 1967, 1970, 1972) the effect of antihypertensive therapy could be demonstrated easily, because patients with high cardiovascular risk and a high incidence of pre-existing cardiovascular events were studied. If trials are conducted in populations with lower risk, however, the number of patients or the duration of the study have to be increased. Treatment of patients with uncomplicated hypertension is a method of primary prevention of coronary heart disease and cerebrovascular accidents. Treatment of uncomplicated hypertension in patients with pre-existing organ damage is a method of secondary prevention. In the latter case more cardiovascular events occur. The number of cardiovascular events is further increased in a population with other risk factors than hypertension.

The well known findings of older intervention trials (Berglund et al. 1978; Veterans Administration, cooperative Study Group on Antihypertensive Aents 1967, 1970, 1972) have not been demonstrated in newer trials. In recent years the HDFP study (1979 a, b, 1982 a, b) and the Australian Trial (1980, 1982; Doyle 1982) have been completed and new data on these trials are still being published. The MRC Trial is also in progress and will hopefully help to clarify many unanswered questions. A summary of trials of the treatment of mild hypertension is given in the WHO/ISH Mild Hypertension Liaison Committee Interim Analysis (1982).

Table 1. 5-Year follow-up of 1943 untreated patients (Australian Therapeutic Trial in Mild Hypertension 1982)

	Percentage
Normotensive	48
No change	32
Increased blood pressure	12
Complications	8

In the HDFP study (1979 a, b, 1982 a, b) no untreated control group was used. Stepped care was compared with referred care. In stepped care patients, blood pressure was slightly lower and cardiovascular events were fewer than in referred care patients. This was true of all blood pressure strata and for all other characteristics studied. There was only one exception of this rule: white women did not appear to benefit from stepped care treatment. In addition, the benefit of stepped care in younger patients (30–49 years) was rather small. (5.7% versus 25.3% in 50–59 year old patients and 16.4% in 60–69 year old patients). There is no proven explanation for these two phenomena. It is possible that compliance in white women is so good that the outcome of referred care could not be improved by stepped care. Stepped care was especially beneficial in patients with diastolic blood pressures of 90–104 mm Hg who had no evidence of end-organ damage and were not receiving treatment when they entered the study (HDFP Study 1982).

In the Australian Trial (1980) treatment significantly reduced cerebrovascular events, but did not affect ischaemic heart disease to any great extent. The Australian Trial generated two additional very important pieces of information. Those patients whose blood pressure was returned to a certain level by treatment had a higher risk of cardiovascular events than patients in the control group who achieved the same pressure without treatment (Doyle 1982). This shows that the degree of benefit does not reach 100% as has been reported for cerebrovascular disease (HDFP Study 1982 b; Trafford et al. 1981) and ischaemic heart disease (Trafford et al. 1981). In fact it would be very suprising if hypertension did not cause irreversible cardiovascular damage before it was treated.

Such damage could only be prevented or reduced by extensive screening for hypertension and by early treatment. The second important impact of the Australian Study concerns untreated mild hypertension (Table 1). The follow-up to that study shows the importance of repeated blood pressure measurement even in mild hypertension. In some ways the new guidelines for mild hypertension of the World Health Organization (WHO 1983.25) are the consequence of the results of the Australian Trial.

Guidelines for the treatment of mild hypertension

The guidelines for treatment of mild hypertension were published by WHO (1983). They were endorsed by the participants of the Third Mild Hypertension Conference held in Switzerland in September 1982. The most important data are given in Fig. 1.

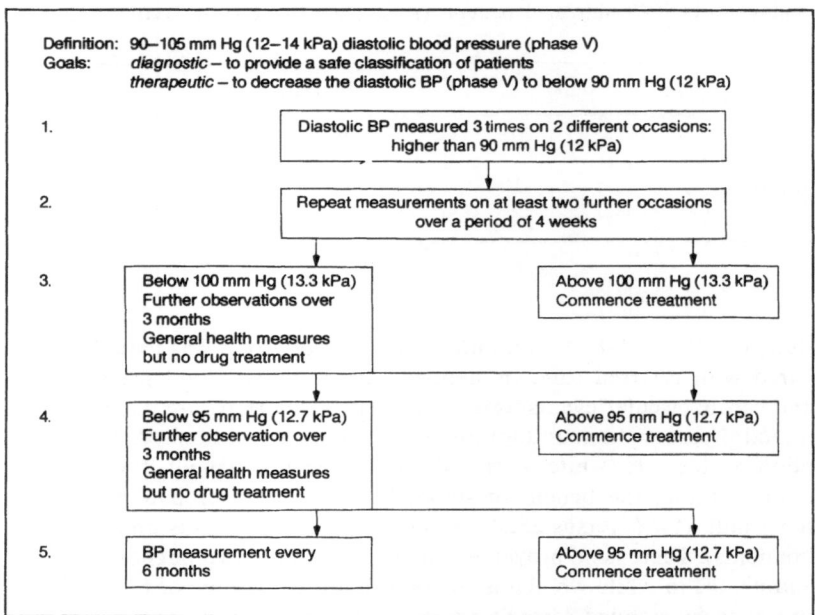

Fig. 1. Definition, blood pressure (BP) measurement and management of mild hypertension. Reproduced, with permission, from Lancet i:457–458 (1983).

The WHO memorandum also mentions other factors influencing the decision for drug treatment. These are listed below.

• A strong family history of cardiovascular disease and an unassociated potentially fatal disease may influence the decision for or against commencement of drug therapy respectively.

• A high systolic blood pressure creates an additional risk for any given diastolic pressure.

• Cardiac signs (clinical, radiological, electro-cardiographic, echocardiographic), unexplained proteinurea, retineal hemorrhage and exudates are all indications for early drug treatment.

• There is no evidence so far that treatment of hypertension in patients over the age of 70 years improves cardiovascular prognosis. Therefore only those patients who are in good health (biological age) should be treated. Patients with debilitating diseases should only be treated if their diastolic pressure consistently exceeds 109 mm Hg. This recommendation is in accordance with preliminary results of the European Working Party on High Blood Pressure in the Elderly (Amery and De Shaepdryver 1981). This group did not find any benefit of treatment in patients over 60 years of age with systolic pressures of 160–239 mm Hg and diastolic pressures of 90–119 mm Hg. Despite these data WHO admits "However, elderly hypertensive patients with cardiac failure benefit significantly from antihypertensive drug treatment".

In addition, compliance of the patient and compatibility of the medication may influence the decision for or against drug treatment in mild hypertension.

Necessity for drug treatment

The general view of the necessity for drug treatment in mild hypertension has become more balanced in recent years (Freis 1982; Kaplan 1983 a, b; McAlister 1983; Morgan 1981; Perry 1982; Pickering 1983) by contrast to the initial response to the HDFP data (Moser 1981). All authors recommend general health measures, the most important of which are weight reduction and salt restriction. It must be kept in mind, however, that obesity is difficult to cure and salt restriction does not reduce blood pressure in the majority of patients. The value of psychological measures has still to be proven. Additionally, avoidance of excess alcohol and cessation of smoking should be recommended. Drug treatment of mild hypertension – as in all other chronic diseases – should be effective, safe, simple, and cheap. In U.S.A., England, France, Italy and Japan, thiazide diuretics are the drugs of first choice, whereas in Germany combinations of diuretics and reserpine or beta-blockers are used most often. After the reports on diuretics in elderly patients (Morgan et al. 1980) and on the effects of beta-blockers on lipid metabolism, (Leren et al 1980), however, these habits have to be questioned. Diuretics cause a prolonged change and beta-blockers a permanent change in lipid metabolism and seem to increase this risk factor in at least some of the patients.

At present there is no concensus on which medication is best in long-term treatment of mild hypertension. Alpha-adrenergic drugs do not influence lipid metabolism adversely. They may even improve the HDL/LDL-ratio (Leren et al. 1980). Alpha-adrenergic drugs have often been accused of causing a high incidence of side-effects but these drugs were primarily used in moderate and severe hypertension. Therefore they were used in high doses and this could explain the high incidence of side-effects. In mild hypertension small doses may be effective and free of subjective and objective side-effects.

Summary

In mild hypertension the decision to treat should be based on repeated blood pressure measurements. Besides general health measures, drug treatment may be neccesary. Side-effects and adverse metabolic effects have to be monitored closely. With this in mind, the role of alpha-adrenergic drugs has to be reconsidered.

References

1 Amery A, De Schaepdryver A (1981) Antihypertensive therapy in patients above age sixty. In: Onesti G, Kim ME (eds) Hypertension in the young and the old. Grune & Stratton, New York, 315–326.
2 Australian Therapeutic Trial in Mild Hypertension (1980) Lancet i: 1261–1267.
3 Australian Therapeutic Trial in Mild Hypertension. Untreated mild hypertension (1982) Lancet i: 185–191.
4 Berglund G, Wilhelmsen L, Sannerstedt R et al. (1978) Coronary heart disease after treatment of hypertension. Lancet i: 1–5.
5 Doyle AE (1982) Australian Therapeutic Trial in Mild Hypertension. Clin Sci 63:431s–434s.
6 Freis ED (1982) Should mild hypertension be treated? N Engl J Med 307:306–309.
7 Hypertension Detection and Follow-up Program Study (1979a) Five-year findings of the hypertension detection and follow-up program. I. Reduction in mortality of persons with high blood pressure, including mild hypertension. JAMA 242:2562–2571.

8 Hypertension Detection and Follow-up Program Study (1979 b) Five-year findings of the hypertension detection and follow-up program. II. Mortality by race-sex and age. JAMA 242:2572–2577.

9 Hypertension Detection and Follow-up Program Study (1982 a) Five-year findings of the hypertension detection and follow-up program. III. Reduction in stroke incidence among persons with high blood pressure. JAMA 247:633–638.

10 Hypertension Detection and Follow-up Program Study (1982 b) The effect of treatment in "mild" hypertension. N Engl J Med 307:976–980.

11 Kaplan NM (1983 a) Mild hypertension. When and how to treat. Arch Int Med 143:255–259.

12 Kaplan NM (1983 b) Therapy for mild hypertension. JAMA 249:365–367.

13 Leren P, Foss PO, Helgeland A, Hjermann I, Holme I, Lund-Larsen PG (1980) Effect of propranolol and prazosin on blood lipids. The Oslo Study. Lancet ii:4–6.

14 McAlister NH (1983) Should we treat mild hypertension? JAMA 249:279–382.

15 Morgan TO (1981) Drug or non-drug therapy for mild hypertension? Curr Ther 50:39–42.

16 Morgan TO, Adam WR, Hodgson M, Gibberd RW (1980) Failure of therapys to improve prognosis in elderly males with hypertension. Med J Austr 2:27–31.

17 Moser M (1981) "Less severe" hypertension: Should it be treated? Am Heart J 101:465–472.

18 Perry HM jr. (1982) Mild hypertension – when and how to treat it. Praxis 71:265–274.

19 Pickering TG (1983) Treatment of mild hypertension and the reduction of cardiovascular mortality: The "of or by'- dilemma. JAMA 249:399–400.

20 Trafford JAP, Horn CR, O'Neal H, McGonigle R, Halford-Maw L, Evans R (1981) Five year follow-up of effects of treatment of mild and moderate hypertension. Br Med J 282:1111–1113.

21 Veterans Administration Cooperative Study Group on Anti-hypertensive Agents (1967) Effects of treatment on morbidity in hypertension. Results in patients with diastolic pressures averaging 115 through 129 mm Hg. JAMA 202:116–122.

22 Veterans Administration Cooperative Study Group on Anti-hypertensive Agents (1970) Effects of treatment on morbidity in hypertension. II. Results in patients with diastolic blood pressure averaging 90 through 114 mm Hg. JAMA 213:1143–1152.

23 Veterans Administration Cooperative Study Group on Anti-hypertensive Agents (1972) Effects of treatment on moribidity in hypertension. III. Influence of age, diastolic pressure and prior cardiovascular disease; further analysis of side effects. Circulation 45:991–1004.

24 WHO/ISH Mild Hypertension Liaison Committee: Trials of the treatment of mild hypertension. An interim analysis. (1982) Lancet i:149–156.

25 WHO (1983) Guidelines for the treatment of mild hypertension: memorandum from a WHO/ISH meeting. Lancet i:457–458.

Correspondence:
K. Hayduk, M. D.
Marien-Hospital
Rochusstraße 2
4000 Düsseldorf 30
F.R.G.

Discussion

MCMAHON:

I think that more emphasis should be given to the treatment of mild hypertension without drugs even though this has not been formally proved to lower morbidity. For instance, hypertension is reduced by modest sodium restriction and by caloric restriction in obese people. I think physical exercise is beneficial and indolence is a risk factor, although probably a mild one. Some of the long-term side-effects of thiazides are the same as those of beta-blockers: beta-blockers have adverse effects on lipids. I believe that the reduction of HDL cholesterol and the elevation of triglycerides are quite well confirmed. I am not sure of the long-term clinical significance of the elevation of uric acid, triglycerides or glucose but I think I am prepared to take the chance on it as thiazides have served us very well since 1955. I have also changed my position on diuretics. I was a little biased because most of my patients are black and they do well with a diuretic. (50–70% of black patients with essential hypertension have an expanded plasma volume). You have to classify the patient in terms of his personality and lifestyle, and whether he is black or white, old or young. All these factors influence which drugs, if any, should be used. At what blood pressure should drugs be started? In patients with a diastolic pressure of 90–95 mm Hg, I watch them for 3 months if there are no other risk factors. If a 35-year-old male has no identifiable risk factor, and his blood pressure is reduced from 165 to 135 mm Hg (the best we can do with an available agent) you change his risk of having cardiovascular disease from 3.5 to 2.5%. This 1% reduction of risk is not worthwhile. On the other hand, if the man is hypercholesterolaemic, smokes cigarettes and has diabetes mellitus you reduce his risk by about 15% and that is worthwhile. One has to treat the other risk factors as well as the hypertension.

KOBINGER:

Why are none of the alpha-stimulating drugs like clonidine or alpha methyl dopa included in the Step 1 treatment?

FRANKLIN:

Our next speaker – Dr Sambhi – is going to address the question of step care therapy.

Current assessment of the stepped-care treatment of mild hypertension: diuretics, beta-blockers, vasodilators versus clonidine

M. P. Sambhi

Introduction

The fairly conclusive demonstration by the Veterans Administration Cooperative Study Group on Antihypertensive Agents (1967) of the strikingly favourable effect of drug treatment on morbidity associated with untreated moderate-to-severe hypertension generated global interest. It suggested that physicians should be made more aware of effective regimens for antihypertensive therapy. A subsequent analysis of the results of the VA trial (Walker et al. 1982) indicated that the benefits of drug treatment, in terms of reducing mortality and morbidity, were, in gross terms, proportional to the therapeutic reduction of blood pressure.

Public health surveys suggested that there were large numbers of untreated hypertensives, and that those under care were often inadequately treated. The teaching of the day emphasized rigorous control of elevated blood pressure. Achievement of goal blood pressure was the prime objective. The benefits of treatment for the vast majority, it was said, far outweighed any risks or inconvenience.

It was against this background that the U.S. Joint National Committee on Detection, Evaluation and Treatment of High Blood Pressure (1980) endorsed the step-care approach. This scheme has the virtue of simplicity and can be understood with ease by the layman.

The step-care approach to the treatment of moderately severe hypertension with multiple drugs incorporates a basic aim of empirical polytherapy, i.e. to achieve a therapeutic effect with minimal toxicity and side-effects. The present report examines whether, as many have suggested, the same simplified approach is suitable for the management of mild hypertension, when the decision in favour of drug treatment has been made.

Implications of step-care treatment of mild hypertension

There are two specific dictates of the step-care approach, as conventionally defined on both sides of the Atlantic which are arguably unsuitable for most, if not all, patients with hypertension.

The first dictate says that even if the initial therapeutic agent, drug A, is ineffective, add drug B to it, and if still required, add another drug, C, to both A and B. The second dictate, which is not stated so tacitly, is that A and B should always be thiazide diuretics or a diuretic and a beta-blocker.

I shall now summarize my reasons for believing that the principles of treating moderately severe hypertension cannot be extended to mild hypertension. Further details can be found elsewhere (Sambhi 1982 and 1983a).

The recently completed trials on mild hypertension discussed by previous speakers have demonstrated that whereas drug treatment in mild hypertension affords significant protection against those complications that are predominantly dependent on the level of elevated blood pressure – namely, cardiac failure and stroke – the influence of drug treatment on morbidity and mortality associated with coronary artery disease is still not clear cut (Sambhi 1983 b).

This situation is particularly important, since the incidence of so-called pressure-dependent complications is rather small in mild hypertension; the major risk associated with it is potentiation of atherosclerosis (Paul 1971) and coronary artery disease, particularly in the male and the post-menopausal female.

Several assumptions and extrapolations commonly made in favour of drug treatment of mild hypertension are unsupportable, and even erroneous. There is, for instance, good evidence from the data accumulated by The Society of Actuaries (1959) and from The Framingham Study (Kannel 1978) that the expected incidence of cardiovascular mortality can be expressed as a linear function of both systolic and diastolic blood pressures. This relationship extends to subnormal levels of blood pressure. It would be a mistake, however, to infer from this evidence that a therapeutically reduced blood pressure can bestow the same cardiovascular status as a physiologically low blood pressure. Indeed, the aggressive lowering of blood pressure in subjects with regional circulatory stenosis carries a well-recognised potential risk.

Another misplaced extrapolation still commonly made is that since we have 25 years experience of treating hypertension with diuretics, and these agents are well tolerated by patients, we should continue to use them as the initial drug for the long-term treatment of mild hypertension. It must be remembered that the experience of 25 years relates to the use of diuretics in the treatment of moderate-to-severe hypertension. As adjuncts to polytherapy, diuretics are undoubtedly an essential ingredient and potentiate the antihypertensive effects of all other agents, but we do not have extensive experience of diuretic monotherapy for the treatment of mild hypertension. Furthermore, to say that thiazide diuretics are the best-tolerated agents is to ignore mounting evidence that they are associated with potentially deleterious metabolic effects (hyperlipidaemia, hyperglycaemia, hyperuricaemia and hypokalaemia) and increase the viscosity of blood (Sambhi 1981).

The work of the Multiple Risk Factor Intervention Trial Research Group (1982), in the U.S.A. has strengthened the notion that diuretic treatment of mild hypertension may have contributed to the increased mortality observed in the treated versus the non-treated groups. Conclusive evidence on the influence of long-term use of a diuretic or a beta-blocker on morbidity and mortality in large numbers of patients with mild hypertension is not available, though the M.R.C. trial nearing completion in the U.K. should yield valuable data.

The matters discussed above emphasize that the benefit/risk ratio for drugs used in the treatment of mild hypertension should not be extrapolated from that for moderate-to-severe hypertension.

I shall now briefly review selected aspects of drugs that can be used as initial agents in monotherapy before proceeding to polytherapy, and later examine how this approach differs from the conventional step-care concept.

Diuretics

The recently published VA cooperative study comparing propranolol with hy-drochlorothiazide (Walker et al. 1982) in the initial treatment of mild hypertension clearly establsihed that the latter is the more effective in the American black, whereas both agents were effective in the white population. Race therefore appears to be an important factor in the choice of these drugs. The results of our own study, shown in Fig. 1, indicate another important, hitherto unrecognized, criterion. This predicts not only whether the antihypertensive response to thiazide diuretics is likely to be optimal or suboptimal, but also indicates whether the elevation in the activity of the renin sys-

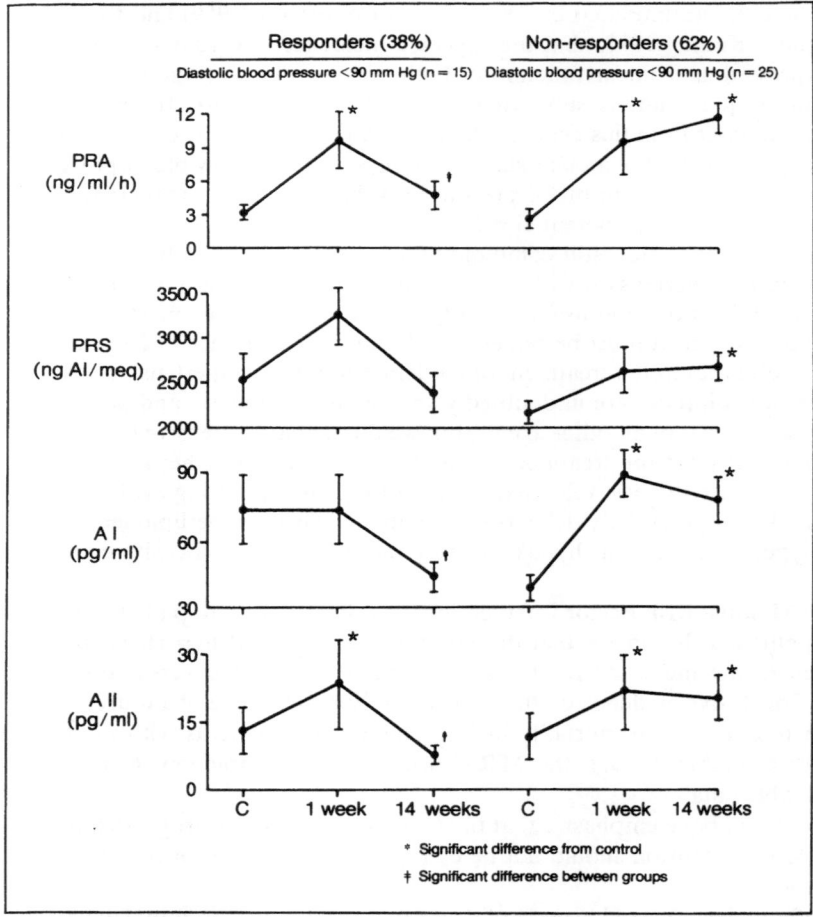

Fig. 1. Forty patients with asymptomatic mild hypertension were treated with hydrochlorothiazide 50 mg. Plasma renin activity (PRA), plasma renin substrate (PRS), blood levels of angiotensin I (AI) and angiotensin II (AII), were all acutely stimulated in all patients. The contrasting behaviour of these parameters during chronic therapy is shown. There was no difference between the two groups at baseline.

tem observed during the acute period of therapy would continue unabated during the chronic phase of treatment.

It is noteworthy that in the so called responders, who achieved goal blood pressure, all of the renin-angiotensin parameters returned to normal values following acute elevation, whereas in the non-responders the values remained significantly elevated. There was no difference between the two groups during the control period. Baseline renin was not a predictor of the subsequent response. All but two of the 25 non-responders showed an abnormal ECG, including either a pattern of left ventricular hypertrophy or non-specific evidence of arteriosclerotic changes in the myocardium. In contrast, only 1 of the 15 responders had electrocardiographic evidence of left ventricular hypertrophy. The implications of these data are fully discussed elsewhere (Sambhi et al. to be published).

Two significant points need to be emphasized. In patients with an abnormal ECG but otherwise uncomplicated mild hypertension, thiazide diuretics may not be the drug of initial choice. Secondly, and equally importantly, it would be unwise to continue the diuretic in the non-responders, as sanctioned by the step-are approach, since this would invite unwanted, long-term adverse consequences, notably in arteriosclerotic heart disease.

The potential of thiazide diuretic therapy to cause hyperlipidaemia has already been referred to, and two recent studies that tend to minimize this effect deserve a brief comment. In the VA cooperative study (Walker et al. 1982) most subjects were black, with significantly lower values for serum triglycerides (genetic or nutritional factors) Furthermore, the standard deviation of all measurements was extremely large. In the Gothenburg study reported by Berglund and Andersson (1981) the patients were carefully and closely followed and given dietary advice. This factor, which was acknowledged by the authors, probably explains why this study did not show serum lipid elevation with prolonged diuretic therapy. The suggestion is strengthened by the preliminary report on the side effects of drugs in the M.R.C. trial (1981) in which, unlike the two studies cited above, there was an untreated control group. The cholesterol elevations, albeit modest, were rendered quite significant because the serum cholesterol had declined in the untreated control group over the same period of time.

Beta-blockers

These agents are suitable and efficacious for many patients but are not free from side-effects (M.R.C. 1981). Most beta-blockers, however, have long-term metabolic effects that resemble those caused by thiazide diuretics, namely hyperglycaemia and hyperuricaemia, together with a lowering of high density lipoproteins and an elevation of low density lipoproteins (Helgeland 1980). There is preliminary evidence (van Brummelen 1983) to suggest that beta-blockers with intrinsic sympathomimetic activity may differ in this respect. It has yet to be discovered whether these metabolic effects of prolonged beta-blocker therapy induce the production of atheroma and neutralize the potential benefits of beta-blockade on the myocardium. It is also not known whether the effect of long-term beta-blocker therapy of reducing blood pressure by reducing cardiac output, without change in peripheral resistance (Lund-Johanson 1979b) is likely to compromise the long-term function of the myocardium. In a ten-year follow-up of those patients with mild hypertension who did not show changes in blood pressure,

Lund-Johanson (1979a) has reported that haemodynamic changes included a reduction in cardiac output and an increase in peripheral resistance. Would it be correct to assume that prolonged beta-blockade does not alter the haemodynamic natural history of early mild hypertension? Again, the results of the M.R.C. trial should provide relevant information, particularly on the question of whether prolonged beta-blockade given to patients with a healthy myocardium has a prophylactic protective action against fatal or non-fatal events associated with ischaemic heart disease.

Vasodilators

Vasodilators with a direct effect on smooth muscle generally result in sodium retention. This action is due to a lowering of pressure natriuresis, and elevation of renin and aldosterone. These agents also activate baroreflex mechanisms which increase sympathetic discharge and stimulate both ionotropic and chronotropic functions of the myocardium, leading to increased cardiac work and oxygen demand. This factor is particularly marked for those vasodilators which predominantly dilate arterioles; not only do they lack the venodilator effect, but they may actually produce venoconstriction. If used alone, these agents can induce angina or myocardial infarction in susceptible patients and are best used in conjunction with a beta-blocker and a diuretic. This is the so-called 'triple therapy' that has proved quite successful in treating moderately severe hypertension. For the treatment of mild hypertension in elderly patients with insensitive baroreceptors, very small doses of hydrallazine alone may be well tolerated.

On the other hand, vasodilators which dilate both arterioles and the venous system act as preload reducers due to venous pooling. By definition, however, these agents should result in volume expansion and sodium retention if used without a diuretic.

Only a brief mention of new agents under evaluation for monotherapy of mild hypertension is appropriate. The currently approved angiotensin-converting enzyme inhibitor, captopril, even at low doses, is beset with relatively infrequent but serious side-effects. M.K. 421 (Merck, Shapr & Dohme) is under evaluation. Only a minority of patients respond to these agents alone, and most require the addition of a diuretic.

Perhaps the most promising class of drugs, albeit still under evaluation, is the heterogeneous group called calcium-channel blockers. If proven safe and effective as antihypertensive agents, these drugs, with demonstrated antianginal and antiarrythmic properties will be the most notable advance in the treatment of mild hypertension. We have preliminary evidence on the saluretic and diuretic properties of one of these agents (Thananopavarn et al. in press).

Clonidine

We have previously described (Sambhi 1983a & b) the features of clonidine that make it a suitable agent for initial therapy, despite the rather high incidence of symptomatic side-effects. These features include a complete lack of metabolic, biochemical or hormonal perturbations. The drug acts predominantly on the central nervous system, stimulating alpha-adrenoceptors linked to peripheral neurons that inhibit blood pressure, heart rate and sympathetic activity. This mechanism has the virtue of not blocking the peripheral sympathetic mediation of reflexes related to posture, exercise and sexual function.

82

Clomerular filtration rate and renal blood flow are unchanged during clonidine therapy (Thananopavarn et al. 1982). In our studies, now confirmed by others, cardiac output remained unchanged and peripheral resistance declined. With significant bradycardia, stroke volume actually increases. Lund-Johansson (1974), however, in earlier careful invasive studies, reported a modest decline in cardiac output after prolonged treatment with clonidine.

Walker et al. (1982) reported a double-blind trial lasting six months, in which clonidine and guanabenz were compared in 188 patients, 61% of whom were classified as mildly hypertensive. Approximately 65% of the patients tolerated and responded well to clonidine monotherapy (dose range 0.1–0.8 mg daily), an additional 6.3% were considered treatment-related dropouts, and the remainder were given a change of therapy or had a diuretic added. The incidence at six months of drowsiness and dry mouth was 26% and

Table 1. Glonidine monotherapy

Recommended regimen for mild hypertension: initial dose and titration schedule

1. Clonidine 0.05 b.i.d. to t.i.d
2. Clonidine 0.05 b.i.d. plus 0.1 mg H.S.
3. Titrate dose upwards:
   a) In small increments
   b) At 2–4-week intervals
   c) Ceiling dose of 0.9 mg
   d) Allow time for symptomatic side effects to diminish or become tolerable
4. If therapeutically optimal dose is not tolerated, reduce the dose and add a small dose of a diuretic or a beta-blocker

Table 2. Clonidine monotherapy

Mild hypertension in elderly
(n = 22–3F; 19 M)

Age: 60–84 yrs.   B.P. < 180/109 mm Hg
Therapeutic goal: diastolic B.P. < 90 mm Hg
(Data from outpatient open trial)

Blood pressure	Control	3 months
Systolic (mm Hg)	172 ± 4	140 ± 4
Diastolic (mm Hg)	106 ± 3	88 ± 2
Required daily dose range	0.1 mg 0.2 0.3 mg 0.4 0.6	3–5 subjects at each dose level
Follow-up at 6 months		a) All subjects maintained B.P. control. b) Addition of a diuretic was required in 3 subjects: in 2 females because of weight gain (5 lbs. each, not necessarily drug related); in one male, clonidine dose had to be reduced below optimal because of drowsiness.

23%, respectively, during clonidine monotherapy. These side-effects were mild and decreased considerably with time.

In our experience the support of a physician is of paramount importance in patient compliance. Our recommendations for the use of clonidine as an initial therapeutic agent are listed in Table 1. Table 2 summarizes our experience with clonidine monotherapy in elderly outpatients who tolerated the drug and were followed for six months. We have previously reported (Thananopavarn, in press) the use of the step-care approach in 33 elderly patients with mild hypertension who were all started on chlorthalidone 25 mg daily. Only eight patients achieved goal blood pressure (diastolic less than 90 mm Hg) with diuretic alone, the remainder doing so with the addition of small doses of clonidine, 0.1–0.3 mg (0.2 mg daily, n = 13) and (0.4–0.6 mg, n = 12).

Recommended modifications in the concept of the step-care approach to the treatment of mild hypertension

Patients with mild hypertension are heterogeneous and have various degrees of risk. Commonly employed drugs for the treatment of asymptomatic patients with mild hypertension, although well tolerated by many, are not free of long-term metabolic consequences. Their effects on the natural history of treated disease are not precisely known. Better and innocuous drugs are needed for the long-term treatment of asymptomatic and uncomplicated hypertension. Drugs such as clonidine, which do not induce significant metabolic, biochemical and haemodynamic deviations, should be considered as step-one therapy, despite the associated higher incidence of symptomatic side-effects.

The benefits and risks of treating mild hypertension with drugs differ considerably from those of moderate-to-severe hypertension. Some of the controversial predictors of drug response, such as hormonal and biochemical profiling prior to treatment, have remained a research tool and have not been helpful in practice. There are other well-recognized factors which determine the therapeutic effects of diuretics and beta-blockers, including the age and race of the patient and existing target organ damage. Diurnal variations of blood pressure and the functional status of the cardiovascular system in response to stress are also promising factors for categorizing patients with mild hypertension.

The dilemma of not doing more harm than good by treating mild hypertension remains. It is imperative, therefore, that an attempt should be made to assess the benefit/risk ratio of different drugs for each patient. An overall recipe should not be sanctioned by recommending the step-care approach. Individualized monotherapy should precede the use of drug combinations. When monotherapy with a particular agent fails to achieve goal blood pressure, it should be substituted by another suitable drug. Individualized polytherapy should be used if single agents are not well tolerated, or goal blood pressure is not achieved. If there is a need to preserve the term 'step-care approach', its meaning and intent should be modified for the treatment of mild hypertension.

References

1 Berglund G, Andersson O (1981) Beta-blockers or diuretics in hypertension? A six year follow-up of blood pressure and metabolic side-effects. Lancet I:744–747.
2 Helgeland A (1980) Treatment of mild hypertension: a five-year controlled drug trial: the Oslo study. Am J Med 69:725–732.

3 Kannel WB (1978) Hypertension, blood lipids and cigarette smoking as co-risk factors for coronary heart disease in mild hypertension: to treat or not to treat. In: Perry HM, Smith WM (eds) NY Acad Sci 304:128–139.
4 Lund-Johansen P (1974) Hemodynamic changes at rest and during exercise in long-term clonidine therapy of essential hypertension. Acta Med Scand 195:111–115.
5 Lund-Johansen P (1979 a) Spontaneous changes in central hemodynamics in essential hypertension – a ten-year follow-up study. In Onesti G, Klimt CR (eds) Hypertension – determinants, complications and intervention. Grune & Stratton, New York, 201–209.
6 Lund-Johansen P (1979 b) Hemodynamic consequences of long-term beta-blocker therapy: a 5-year follow-up study of atenolol. J Cardiovasc Pharmacol 1:487–495.
7 MRC (1981) Report of Medical Research Council working party on mild to moderate hypertension: adverse reactions to bendrofluazide and propranolol for the treatment of mild hypertension. Lancet II:539–542.
8 Multiple Risk Factor Intervention Trial Research Group (1982) Multiple risk intervention trial. JAMA 248:1465–1477.
9 Paul O (1971) Risks of mild hypertension: a ten-year report. Br Heart J (Suppl) 33:116–121.
10 Report of the Joint National Committee on detection, evaluation, and treatment of high blood pressure (1980) Arch Intern Med 140:1280–1285.
11 Sambhi MP (1981) The effectiveness of diuretics in hypertension: a critical evaluation. In: Weber MA (ed), Treatment strategies in hypertension. Symposia Specialists, Miami 97–109.
12 Sambhi MP (1982) Individualized drug therapy: a rational alternative to the stepped-care approach in treatment of mild hypertension. International Symposium on Mild Hypertension, Mexico City. In press.
13 Sambhi MP (1983 a) Clonidine monotherapy in mild hypertension. Chest (Suppl 2) 83:427–430.
14 Sambhi MP (1983 b) Clonidin-monotherapie bei leichter und mittelschwerer hypertonie. In: Hayduk K (Hrsg), Bock KD Zentrale Blutdruckregulation durch α_2-Rezoptorenstimulation. Steinkopff Verlag Darmstadt, Düsseldorf, Essen:132–143.
15 Sambhi MP, Thananopavarn C, Eggena P, Berrett JD, to be published.
16 Society of Actuaries (1959) Build and blood pressure study, Chicago, 1.
17 Taguchi J, Freis ED (1974) Partial reduction of blood pressure and prevention of complications in hypertension. Engl J Med 291:329–331.
18 Than nopavarn C, Golub MS, Eggena P, Barrett JD, Sambhi MP (1982) Clonidine, a centrally acting sympathetic inhibitor, as monotherapy for mild to moderate hypertension. Am J Cardiol 49:153–157.
19 Thananopavarn C, Sambhi MP, Golub MS, Eggena P, Barrett JD (March, in press) Saluretic and diuretic effects of nitrendipine during antihypertensive monotherapy. Abstract: Amer Soc Clinic Pharmacol Therap.
20 Thananopavarn C, Golub MS, Sambhi MP (1983) Clonidine in the elderly hypertensive. Monotherapy and therapy with a diuretic. Chest 83 (Suppl):410–411.
21 Van Brummelen P (1983) The relevance of intrinsic sympathomimetic activity for β-blocker-induced changes in plasma lipids. J Cardiovasc Pharmacol 5 (Suppl 1):S51–S55.
22 Veterans Administration Cooperaive Study Group on antihypertensive agents (1967) Effects of treatment on morbidity in hypertension: results in patients with diastolic blood pressures averaging 115 through 129 mm Hg. JAMA 202:116–122.
23 Walker BR, Hare LE, Dwitch MW (1982) Comparative antihypertensive effects of guanabenz and clonidine. J Int Med Res 10:6–14.

Correspondence:
Professor M. P. Sambhi
Division of Hypertension
Department of medicine, UCLA
San Fernando Valley Medical Center
16111 Plummer Street
Sepulveda, California 91343, USA

Discussion

FRANKLIN:
The response to beta-blockade in a hypertensive population suggests the existence of two sub-populations – one that may respond to very low dose therapy and one that will not respond to very high dose therapy, despite a similar reduction in cardiac output. Do you have any thoughts on the mechanisms that may be playing a role here?

SAMBHI:
This is the age-old question – how do beta-blockers work? None of us know but in my experience, most patients who show blood pressure reduction with beta-blockade also show some reduction in cardiac output. Perhaps there is a long-term haemodynamic adjustment, involving beta-receptors, which is responsible for the fall in blood pressure. It cannot be an exclusively central effect, as there are effective beta-blockers which do not cross the blood-brain barrier. It cannot be renin suppression alone as there is no correlation between plasma renin levels and the blood pressure response.

WEBER:
Most of us would agree with the overall approach that Dr Sambhi proposed. I think that we have become disillusioned with step care and with any approach that does not allow us to tailor treatment to the individual. To be fair, beta-blockers have been very useful drugs for the last 10 years. The experience in the United States, of course, is not quite as long as it has been in Europe but I still think that they form a mainstay of treatment. A large number of patients, particularly younger patients, find them very acceptable. Apart from some of the metabolic difficulties alluded to by Dr Sambhi, many young people are keen on physical exercise such as running or tennis and beta-blockers may severely impair the ability to perform vigorous physical activities. This causes a problem for some younger patients. A monotherapy, preferably not a diuretic, is needed which will reduce blood pressure in young people without reducing exercise tolerance. Whether cloni-dine or converting enzyme inhibitors will fulfill these criteria, I am not sure, but I do not think that beta-blockers are a universal answer.

SAMBHI:
We also have several young patients, who were on beta-blockers and complained that they could not take part in the competitive sports that they used to.

PEART:
I think that there is little doubt that the response is variable. I do not think that the metabolic handling of beta-blockers is understood. The oldest of them – propranolol – is affected by first-pass metabolism which contributes to the response variability and may lie behind some of the dos-age variability observed in subjects on propranolol. The dose may have to be varied as much as five-fold to produce a given effect, even on the heart rate. The biological effect lasts much longer than any drug levels in plasma and the disposition and action of the drug at different sites are still unclear. Some think that atenolol does not enter the brain but I am quite sure that it does, my patients tell me that it does and I trust what they say. The other problem is the muscular effect; this is one reason why such patients cannot perform strenuous exercise. The sensation in the muscle is a very variable feature. There is also the effect on respiration which is worse with pro-pranolol but exists with all beta-blockers. The more exercise is possible, the more it is likely that inability to breathe properly will be noted. There are lots of minus factors to beta-blocker therapy which must be put into the equation before a decision is made to start to treat mild hypertension.

SAMBHI:
Professor Peart, you have long experience of the use of beta-blockers in the UK. What do you think of those with intrinsic sympathomimetic activity? Do they have advantages?

PEART:
It is claimed that it is beneficial to use beta-blockers which have intrinsic activity because the heart is not slowed down as much as by those which do not. There is no hard evidence of this benefit.

HAYDUK:

Two remarks. First, diuretics do not reduce exercise blood pressure as much as beta-blockers do; to what extent does clonidine reduce exercise blood pressure? Second, I have a comment. In Germany we do not like to combine beta-blockers and clonidine.

SAMBHI:

I do not have any personal experience with clonidine in exercise but I think from the studies of others that it does not decrease ability as much as the beta-blockers do. I think that I can recall a study in which the exercise blood pressure was reduced quite effectively with clonidine.

DRAYER:

You said in your lecture that non-responders to diuretics more often had left ventricular hypertrophy as revealed by the electrocardiogram (or the MRFIT definition of an abnormal electrocardiogram). They had the same baseline blood pressure and they were more or less the same age so there were no specific reasons why that group had a more abnormal electrocardiogram. Do they have longer standing hypertension? Then do you have any reason for this phenomenon?

SAMBHI:

It was a retrospective analysis, of course, in terms of the electrocardiogram but obviously in the same age group you can have myocardial dysfunction as a result of a variety of causes or you can have a healthy myocardium. The group divided itself into these strikingly different sections. We went back and looked into whether there were any other differences we could define: age, duration of high blood pressure, the severity of the pressure or plasma renin. There were none and we were unable to distinguish these people by their renin profiles.

Use of centrally-acting agonists in the treatment of mild hypertension in the elderly patient

J. I. M. Drayer, M. A. Weber

The treatment of patients with mild hypertension has created considerable interest in recent years. The availability of many potent antihypertensive agents allows blood pressure to be effectively controlled without major adverse effects. It is believed that control of even mild elevations of blood pressure significantly reduces the incidence of major cardiovascular complications.

It is now well accepted that both systolic and diastolic hypertension are direct risk factors for cardiovascular complications (Kannel 1974; Kannel et al. 1979). This finding is particularly relevant to the elderly population. Systolic blood pressure in elderly hypertensive patients is often more clearly elevated than diastolic blood pressure. Many elderly patients have predominant or isolated systolic hypertension. In these elderly patients systolic blood pressure is usually greater than 150 mm Hg and diastolic blood pressure less than 100 mm Hg.

One should recognize that the elevated blood pressure seen in these patients is often not the only cardiovascular risk factor. The incidence of atherosclerotic heart disease increases with age as does the incidence of arrhythmias and cardiac hypertrophy. Moreover, diabetes mellitus is a common disease in the elderly population (Barrett-Connor et al. 1981). By contrast, obesity and cigarette smoking are risk factors more often found in younger than in older patients (Stebbins et al. 1981).

Recent studies have shown that the presence of cardiovascular risk factors are important in determining the choice of antihypertensive agents. Monotherapy with diuretics might be harmful in patients with an increased risk of cardiovascular disease. In these patients, monotherapy with other antihypertensive agents such as sympatholytic drugs should be considered.

Characteristics of patients with systolic hypertension

It is believed that the increase in systolic blood pressure in the elderly patient results from decreased elasticity of the aorta and large arteries. When blood pressure increases in these patients it expresses itself as elevated systolic rather than diastolic blood pressure. By contrast, in patients with a normal vascular bed hypertensive mechanisms induce elevations of both systolic and diastolic blood pressure. Indeed, increases in diastolic blood pressure are more clearly seen in young patients and increases in systolic blood pressure prevail in the older population (Drayer et al. 1981).

We have argued previously (Drayer et al. 1982) that hypertension in the elderly is not necessarily a consequence of long-standing disease. In a group of 74-year-old hypertensive patients the duration of the disease was only 11 years, compared with 8 years in 46-year-old hypertensives. The average blood pressure in the younger group

Table 1. Clinical characteristics of patients with systolic and diastolic hypertension

	Systolic hypertension (n = 200)	Probability p	Diastolic hypertension (n = 419)
Systolic blood pressure (mm Hg)	168 ± 14	ns	170 ± 24
Diastolic blood pressure (mm Hg)	90 ± 8	< 0.001	108 ± 9
Age (years)	56 ± 13	< 0.001	49 ± 11
Duration of hypertension (years)	9 ± 10	ns	9 ± 9
Relative body weight (%)	123 ± 26	ns	122 ± 22
Sex ratio (% women)	52	< 0.001	37

ns = not significant

was 150/101 mm Hg compared with 176/92 mm Hg in the elderly patients. It is unlikely that the difference of 26 mm Hg in systolic blood pressure is a consequence of the slightly longer duration of the disease in the older population. In a further analysis of the data (Drayer et al. submitted) a group of 619 hypertensive patients with essential hypertension was subdivided into those with predominant systolic hypertension (seated systolic blood pressure greater than 150 mm Hg and diastolic blood pressure less than 100 mm Hg, n = 200) and those with diastolic hypertension (seated diastolic blood pressure greater than 99 mm Hg, n = 419). Diastolic blood pressures were significantly different between the two groups but systolic blood pressures were quite similar (Table 1). The patients with predominant systolic hypertension were further characterized by a greater fall in systolic blood pressure (−8 ± 14 vs −3 ± 15 mm Hg, p < 0.01) and a smaller increase in diastolic blood pressure (+ 1 ± 8 vs + 3 ± 9 mm Hg, not significant) when they assumed the upright posture.

The duration of high blood pressure was similar for both groups, as was the degree of obesity. Patients with systolic hypertension were slightly older than patients with diastolic hypertension, and women were more often found among patients with systolic hypertension than among those with diastolic hypertension. Evidence of end organ damage related to the elevated blood pressure, such as clinically significant changes found during fundoscopic examination or electrocardiographic evidence for left ventricular hypertrophy, were similar in the two groups. Moreover, signs of atherosclerotic disease, such as the presence of a strain pattern or signs of an old myocardial infarction on the electrocardiogram, were equally common in patients with systolic hypertension and those with diastolic hypertension (Table 2).

The aetiology of hypertension in the elderly

The aetiology of systolic hypertension is not well known. Some investigators have shown that sodium retention may occur in elderly patients as a result of the age-related decrease in kidney function (Beretta-Piccoli et al. 1982). In other patients, enhanced

Table 2. Evidence for cardiovascular disease in patients with systolic and diastolic hypertension

	Systolic hypertension (n=200)	Probability p	Diastolic hypertension (n=419)
Incidence of fundoscopic changes – Grade 2 or 3 (%)	25	ns	27
QRS voltage in chest leads (mm)	29±8	ns	29±9
Incidence of strain pattern on ECG (%)	30	ns	26
Incidence of old myocardial infarction of ECG (%)	17	ns	11

ns = not significant

sodium excretion with harmful hyponatraemia has been observed (Ashraf et al. 1981). In our study we did not find a significant difference between the blood pressures of patients who excreted low amounts of sodium in their urine (less than 70 meq/g creatinine/24 hours) and those who had a high dietary sodium intake with urinary sodium excretion rates greater than 100 meq/g creatinine/24 hours (167/90 vs 169/91 mm Hg, not significantly different). Similarly, blood pressure levels did not correlate significantly with sodium excretion rates in patients with diastolic hypertension.

Low levels of plasma renin activity are more often found in older patients or in those with systolic hypertension than in younger patients or patients with diastolic hypertension. Moreover, aldosterone excretion rates do not decrease with age to the same extent as plasma renin activity. Thus, the aldosterone:renin ratio increases with age. These changes might promote mild sodium retention in elderly hypertensive patients (Drayer et al. 1981). Indeed, elderly patients with low renin hypertension respond particularly well to treatment with a diuretic (Niarchos 1980).

Catecholamine levels tend to be slightly higher in older patients (Bühler et al. 1982; Messerli et al. 1981a). The pressor response to noradrenaline increases with age (Palmer et al. 1978). Thus, increased activity of the sympathetic nervous system or an increased response to sympathomimetic stimuli might play a role in the aetiology of mild systolic and/or diastolic hypertension in the elderly. Increased sympathetic stimulation may cause an increase in blood pressure due to stimulation of alpha-adrenergic receptors in the smooth muscle cells of the vascular wall. In turn, stimulation of these receptors will increase vasoconstriction which will not entirely be offset by simultaneous stimulation of peripheral beta-2-receptors. Indeed, the number of beta-receptors decreases with age (Schocken & Roth 1977).

Hypertension in the elderly patient might also be due to the atherosclerotic changes often found in the arterioles at this age. Atherosclerosis of the small arteries is expected to cause increases in diastolic blood pressure. Therefore, atherosclerosis might be a factor in elderly patients with diastolic hypertension. It has been shown that the incidence of hypertension in patients with atherosclerotic cardiovascular complications i.e. ischaemic heart disease) is not greater than expected in the adult population (Norwegian Multicentre Study Group, 1981).

Treatment of mild systolic and diastolic hypertension in the elderly

It is obvious from the previous discussion that a clear understanding of the mechanisms involved in the development of hypertension in elderly patients has not been obtained. It seems apparent that most evidence suggests a plausible role for increased sympathetic nervous system activity in the aetiology of this form of hypertension. In addition, a subgroup of these patients might be characterized by a slightly increased sodium retention. Only a few studies have been done to relate these aetiological considerations to therapy.

Niarchos (1980) has treated elderly hypertensive patients with diuretics and with the beta-adrenergic blocking agent, propranolol. He found that diuretics were effective, especially in elderly patients with hypertension and a low plasma renin activity. Propranolol was more often effective in elderly patients with normal renin hypertension. Low renin levels are relatively common and high renin relatively rare in the elderly. Thus, diuretics might be a good first choice in elderly hypertensives. However, disadvantages of this approach include that overt signs of ischaemic heart disease, arrhythmia and/or cardiac hypertrophy are present in a significant number of elderly patients (Kannel et al. 1979). Diuretics have been shown to be harmful in these patients. The use of diuretics in patients with mild hypertension and electrocardiographic abnormalities resulted in an increased rate of cardiovascular events (Multiple Risk Factor Intervention Trial Research Group 1982). Diuretics might induce severe symptomatic hyponatraemia in some elderly hypertensive patients (Ashraf et al. 1981).

Beta-adrenergic blocking agents have been shown to be effective in subgroups of elderly patients with systolic or diastolic hypertension. Propranolol did not lower blood pressure in patients with low-renin forms of systolic or diastolic hypertension. By contrast, elderly patients with normal renin hypertension responded favourably to beta-blocker therapy (Niarchos 1980). Bühler et al. (1975) have shown that the anti-hypertensive effect of propranolol decreases significantly with age. This diminished responsiveness is probably due to the increased incidence of low-renin hypertension in the elderly population.

Centrally-acting, alpha-adrenergic sympatholytic agents are being used with increasing frequency in elderly patients with hypertension. Thananopavarn et al. (1983) were able to control blood pressure with low doses of clonidine (0.1–0.6 mg once or twice daily) in 12 of 15 elderly patients with diastolic hypertension. Low doses of diuretics were needed to achieve blood pressure control in the remaining three patients. In another series of patients, therapy was begun with a low dose of diuretic (25 mg chlorthalidone daily). Therapy with the diuretic resulted in control of blood pressure in only 8 of 33 patients. In the remaining 25 patients, clonidine (0.2 –0.6 mg daily) had to be added to control blood pressure. Thus, in the elderly hypertensive subject initial therapy with clonidine was more effective than monotherapy with a diuretic. Messerli et al. (1981 b) have also shown that therapy with alpha-methyldopa significantly reduces blood pressure in elderly patients with systolic hypertension. The powerful antihypertensive effect of monotherapy with centrally-acting sympatholytic agents such as clonidine and alpha-methyldopa in the elderly supports the important role of the sympathetic nervous system in the aetiology of this form of hypertension.

We have shown recently (Weber et al. 1983) that blood pressure in patients with isolated systolic hypertension can easily be controlled with a combination of a low dose of chlorthalidone (15 mg daily) and clonidine (0.1 mg per day). This combination given once a day controlled blood pressures in 11 of 13 patients. In the remaining two patients the chlorthalidone/clonidine combination was given twice daily. Supine blood pressures fell significantly ($p < 0.01$) in the group as a whole from $170\pm4/93\pm3$ to $141\pm3/81\pm3$ mm Hg. Upright pressures decreased from $172\pm4/93\pm3$ to $135\pm4/85\pm3$ mm Hg ($p < 0.01$). The results of this study reveal that low-dose therapy is highly effective in elderly hypertensive patients. In these patients blood pressure can be controlled without inducing orthostatic changes in blood pressure. Messerli et al. (1981 b) have shown that alpha-methyldopa lowers blood pressure and noradrenaline levels in elderly patients with systolic hypertension, but despite these changes, the cardiovascular responses to change in body position remained intact.

The vasodilatory agent, hydralazine, has also been shown to be effective in elderly hypertensive patients. It can be used as additional therapy for the few patients who do not respond adequately to a diuretic/sympatholytic combination, or it can be administered directly with a diuretic. In older patients this combination does not induce the marked tachycardia observed in younger patients with hypertension. Calcium channel blockers may be used as an alternative to hydralazine.

Conclusions

Many recent publications have focused on the evaluation and therapy of elderly patients with systolic or diastolic hypertension. The data presented suggest that systolic hypertension in this population is a significant risk factor for cardiovascular complications. The cardiovascular status of these patients is often compromised by concomitant ischaemic heart disease and the presence of cardiovascular risk factors such as diabetes mellitus.

The development of hypertension in elderly patients results in increased systolic rather than diastolic blood pressure. Patients with isolated systolic hypertension are characterized by relatively normal diastolic blood pressures and slight but significant orthostatic changes in pressure. This subgroup of patients includes a relatively high percentage of women. Evidence of blood-pressure-related end organ damage and signs of ischaemic heart disease in this subgroup are as common as in patients with diastolic hypertension.

The aetiology of hypertension in the elderly is unknown. Mild sodium retention might play a role in some patients, especially in those with a low plasma renin activity and relatively high excretion rates of aldosterone.

Increased activity of the sympathetic nervous system is likely to cause hypertension in many elderly patients with systolic or diastolic hypertension. Patients with this form of hypertension reveal an enhanced response to pressor stimuli and a marked response of their blood pressure to treatment with centrally acting sympatholytic agents such as clonidine or alpha-methyldopa. In view of the possible harmful effects of diuretic therapy and the marked response to sympatholytic therapy, it seems preferable to start with monotherapy using the centrally-acting sympatholytic agents and to add low doses of a diuretic if blood pressure is not controlled. Vasodilatory drugs may be added if blood pressure is not normalized during combined diuretic/sympatholytic therapy. Thus, systolic or diastolic hypertension may be treated with low doses of specific antihypertensive drugs. However, it remains to be shown that chronic antihypertensive therapy significantly reduces the high rates of mortality and morbidity in these patients.

Summary

Elevated systolic blood pressure is now considered a major risk factor for cardiovascular disease. Isolated or predominant systolic hypertension is more often present in older than in younger patients. Data are presented in this paper which suggest that systolic hypertension has a greater age of onset than diastolic hypertension, and does not develop as a consequence of it. Patients with systolic hypertension are women more often than men. Cardiovascular abnormalities such as signs of hypertensive vascular disease or signs of ischaemic heart disease are as often found in patients with systolic hypertension as in patients with diastolic hypertension.

The aetiology of hypertension in the elderly is not well known. Sodium intake is not clearly related to blood pressure in these patients and diuretic therapy often does not control hypertension in the elderly. It is more likely that an increase in sympathetic nervous system activity is involved in the maintenance of hypertension in these patients. Indeed, therapy with low doses of centrally-acting sympatholytic agents such as clonidine or alpha-methyldopa, alone or in combination with a low dose of a diuretic, has been shown to decrease blood pressure markedly in elderly patients with systolic or diastolic hypertension. However, it remains to be shown that chronic antihypertensive therapy will significantly reduce the high morbidity and mortality rate in the elderly.

References

1 Ashraf N, Locksley R, Arieff AI (1981) Thiazide-induced hyponatraemia associated with death or neurologic damage in outpatients. Am J Med 70:1163–1168.
2 Barrett-Connor E, Criqui MH, Klauber MR, Holdbrook M (1981) Diabetes and hypertension in a community of older adults. Am J Epidemiol 113:276–284.
3 Beretta-Piccoli C, Davies DL, Boddy K et al (1982) Relation of arterial pressure with body sodium, body potassium and plasma potassium in essential hypertension. Clin Sci 63:257–270.
4 Bühler FR, Burkart F, Lütold BE, Küng M, Marbet G, Pfisterer M (1975) Antihypertensive beta-blocking action as related to renin and age: a pharmacologic tool to identify pathogenetic mechanisms in essential hypertension. Am J Cardiol 36:653–669.
5 Bühler FR, Kiowski W, Landmann R et al. (1982) Changing role of beta- and alpha-adrenoreceptor-mediated cardiovascular responses in the transition from high-cardiac output into a high-peripheral resistance phase in essential hypertension. In: Largh JH, Bühler F, Seldin D (Eds.) Frontiers in Hypertension Research, Springer-Verlag, New York, 316–326.
6 Drayer JIM, Weber MA, Laragh JH, Sealey JE (1982) Renin subgroups in essential hypertension. Clin Exp Hypertens A4:1817–1834.
7 Drayer JIM, Weber MA, Sealey JE, Laragh JH (1981) Low and high renin essential hypertension: a comparison of clinical and biochemical characteristics. Am J Med Sci 281:135–142.
8 Drayer JIM, Weber MA, Sealey JE, Laragh JH (submitted for publication 1983). Comparison of clinical characteristics of patients with systolic and diastolic hypertension.
9 Kannel WB (1974) Role of blood pressure in cardiovascular morbidity and mortality. Prog Cardiovasc Dis 17:5–24.

10 Kannel WB, Dawber TR, McGee DL (1980) Perspectives on systolic hypertension. The Framingham Study. Circulation 61:1179–1182.
11 Kannel WB, Gordon T, Castelli WP, Margolis JR (1970) Electrocardiographic left ventricular hypertrophy and risk of coronary heart disease. The Framingham Study. Ann Intern Med 72:813–822.
12 Messerli FH, Gerald MD, Dreslinski GR (1981 b) Antiadrenergic therapy: special aspects in hypertension in the elderly. Hypertension 3 (Suppl II): 226–239.
13 Messerli FH, Glade LB, Dreslinski GR et al (1981 a) Hypertension in the elderly: haemodynamic, fluid volume and endocrine findings. Clin Sci 61:393 s–394 s.
14 Multiple Risk Factor Intervention Trial Research Group (1982) Multiple risk factor intervention trial. Risk factor changes and mortality, results. JAMA 2481:1465–1477.
15 Niarchos AP (1980) Pathophysiology, diagnosis, and treatment of hypertension in the elderly. Cardiovasc Rev Rep 1:621–627.
16 Norwegian Multicenter Study Group (1981) Timolol-induced reduction in mortality and re-infarction in patients surviving acute myocardial infarction. N Engl J Med 304:801–807.
17 Palmer GJ, Ziegler MG, Lake CR (1978) Response of norepinephrine and blood pressure to stress increases with age. J Gerontol 33:482–487.
18 Schocken DD, Roth GS (1977) Reduced beta-adrenergic receptor concentrations in aging man. Nature 267:856–865.
19 Stebbins PT, Taylor GJ, Gibson RS, Beller GA (1980) Risk factors and myocardial infarction in the elderly. Circulation 62 (Suppl III): 220–230.
20 Thananopavarn C, Golub MS, Sambhi MP (1983) Clonidine in the elderly hypertensive. Monotherapy and therapy with a diuretic. Chest 2 (Suppl):410–411.
21 Weber MA, Drayer JIM, Gray DR (1983) Combined diuretic and sympatholytic therapy in elderly patients with predominant systolic hypertension. Chest 2 (Suppl):416–419.

Correspondence:
J. I. M. Drayer, M.D.
Hypertension Center WI30
VA Medical Center
5901 East Seventh Street
Long Beach, CA 90822 USA
213/498–6892

Discussion

MANCIA:
You said that elderly hypertensive subjects have higher sympathetic tone which may contribute to the hypertension but I wonder about the evidence for this. Studies by Reid indicate that the receptor specificity and/or sensitivity of the alpha-receptors does not change with age. Also, I think that we have to look carefully at the plasma noradrenaline concentrations in the elderly. There is a recent paper by Esler which provides evidence that the raised noradrenaline concentration in the elderly may be due to reduced clearance, possibly due to reduced cardiac output and might not have anything to do with an increased secretion rate.

DRAYER:
Your point is taken. The number of alpha-receptors probably does not change with age. If at the same time the number of beta-receptors decreased, however, there might be an over-reactive vasoconstrictor response, but there is little hard evidence for that. Palmer subjected people of different ages to the pressor test and found that the increase in blood pressure is more marked in elderly people than in younger people. The catecholamine data are difficult to interpret but treatment used to block sympathetic activity is apparently quite effective in this group. It is something we have to work at a little more.

TUCK:
We have studied plasma catecholamines in some elderly subjects. There was quite a range but some subjects had remarkably high levels. I do not think that this is explained by clearance although we have not formally examined that possibility. In addition to receptor reduction with increased age, there is a reduction in the adenylate cyclase response and probably the guanidine nucleotide. There is no doubt about that. In select cases that may be contributing to hypertension.

FRANKLIN:
Dr Polinsky, have there been any recent studies at the National Institutes of Health on catecholamine metabolism in the elderly?

POLINSKY:
None that I know of There are some alpha-receptor binding studies in progress and the greatest difference is between males and females but I am not aware that these studies have shown changes as a function of age.

MCMAHON:
I would like to ask a question on the frequency of systolic hypertension in the aged. Gifford stated that one third of all hypertension in patients over the age of 60 or 65 years was systolic hypertension but we attempted to perform a study of hypertension in which blood pressure had to be 160/90 mm Hg and the age had to be over 65 years. We had to screen a huge number of people to find a few who fulfilled the criteria.

DRAYER:
I think you are right. It depends on how you define it and what you want. I think arbitrarily to put the age at 65 years excludes many 50-year-olds who have systolic hypertension. If systolic hypertension is being examined the study should include all ages with a further analysis of the effect of age. Using your definition we have found five such patients in the last four years. The stricter your criteria the harder they are to satisfy. The same is true of young patients with hyperadrenergic syndrome who develop hypertension; I have only seen a few.

HAYDUK:
You showed a significant drop in blood pressure but no change in pulse rate during clonidine treatment. Do you believe that the pulse rate did not drop because the dose was so small or do you believe that older people behave differently?

DRAYER:
It is claimed that older people have a lower heart rate which is harder to stimulate by standing up or by other stimuli, but in this study the dose was extremely low and that is why we did not see much of a change. Nevertheless the heart rate was fairly high anyway. There was no difference in heart rate between the systolic hypertension and the diastolic hypertension groups and in systolic hypertensives below and over 60 years of age. Obviously there are some older people with a low heart rate who will not change their heart rate on standing, who will not change their heart rate with a beta-blocker, who will not change their heart rate with hydralazine, but this is not true of all old people, in my experience.

Sympathetic nervous system activity in the obese hypertensive patient: potential role for central alpha-adrenoreceptor agonists

M. Tuck

The relationship between body weight and blood pressure

In most industrialized populations a strong association between blood pressure and body weight has been established. Several large-scale studies in the United States have confirmed the relationship between obesity and hypertension (the Framingham Study (Kannel et al. 1967); the Evans Country, Georgia Study (Tyroler et al. 1975); the Community Hypertension Evaluation Clinic (Stamler et al. 1978); Hypertensive Detection and Follow-up Program Cooperative Group (1979)). In the Evans county, Georgia study it was demonstrated prospectively that weight gain can increase blood pressure. Over the six-year period of the study, weight gain was associated with a two-fold possibility of developing hypertension. The converse was also true: subjects who were hypertensive at outset gained more weight. In those who were both obese and hypertensive at the outset, a weight reduction programme averaging 8 kg per patient produced very pronounced decrements in both systolic and diastolic blood pressure over a year. Comparing black and white subjects, it was concluded that obese white hypertensives benefited more than blacks from weight loss.

Amongst the million people screened in the Community Hypertension Evaluation Clinic Study, hypertension was two to three times more common in overweight subjects, especially between the ages of 20 and 39 years (Stamler et al. 1978). This relationship was further documented by the Hypertensive Detection and Follow-up Program , Cooperative Group (1979), which showed that 60% of participants chosen for having mild hypertension were also 20% above ideal body weight.

The Framingham Study has yielded important information on the relationships between age, the onset of obesity and changes in blood pressure (Kannel et al. 1979; Gordon and Kannel 1976). The results show that weight is related to blood pressure most strongly in persons under the age of 20 years; as age increases the relationship weakens, especially for diastolic blood pressure. The offspring of the original cohort in the Framingham Study also demonstrated a stronger relation between weight and blood pressure in early adulthood, especially in men (Kannel and Gordon 1968). Other smaller studies have shown that overweight children and adolescents already show higher blood pressure levels than their non-obese counterparts (McCue et al. 1979; Lynds et al. 1980), implying that weight-related blood pressure elevation can begin early in life. In fact, Schacter and co-workers (1982) have noted a significant correlation between weight and blood pressure during the first two years of life. The importance of minimizing weight gain at certain critical periods of life, such as young adulthood, have been emphasized in the prevention of subsequent hypertension (Havlik et al. 1983).

Longitudinal studies have provided further evidence that weight changes can alter blood pressure. The Framingham Study, for example, followed its initial cohorts prospectively and observed that a 10% increase in weight between examinations was accompanied by a 7 mm Hg increase in systolic blood pressure (Ashley and Kannel 1974). In a 30-year follow-up of initially thin, normotensive aviators, those within the upper limits of systolic blood pressure at the end of the study were also the ones who gained the most weight (Harlan et al. 1973). An almost linear relationship between weight and blood pressure could be implied from these studies. But several additional variables such as age, race, sex, types of obesity, methods of measuring obesity and blood pressure, together with family and environmental factors all enter into a seemingly simple relationship.

Bergland et al. (1982) have compared the type of obesity and the incidence of associated hypertension. Body cell mass and fat cell number were unrelated to blood pressure but fat cell size (hypertrophic obesity) was positively correlated. In a careful measurement of body composition and fat cell properties, including underwater weighing and fat cell biopsy, blood pressure correlated best with total body fat mass and fat cell number but not lean body mass or fat cell size (Siervogel et al. 1982). It is also not clear whether skin-fold thickness or body weight is the better predictor of blood pressure. Simple measurements of waist girth may be as good a predictor of blood pressure as more complicated parameters (Berglund et al. 1982). It is also important to bear in mind cuff size. A recent study has re-emphasized the need to measure arm circumference in obese subjects and to use an appropriate cuff size (Maxwell et al. 1982). The use of the regular cuff, it was suggested, may have led to an overestimation of the prevalence of hypertension in obese subjects. There may also be differential effects of obesity on blood pressure. A 32-year follow-up of young men indicated that increased body weight led to higher blood pressure, but it affected systolic pressures more than diastolic (Gillum et al. 1982).

Cardiovascular risk of obesity and hypertension

It is clear that obesity, either directly or indirectly, is a major risk factor for cardiovascular disease. The Framingham Study showed that, in comparison with subjects of normal weight, overweight subjects are four times more likely to have coronary artery disease, as manifested by angina pectoris and sudden death, and seven times more likely to have a stroke (Kannel et al. 1967). Hypertension in obese subjects appeared to be the most likely factor in these cardiovascular conditions. The Framingham Study has also suggested, however, that obesity itself may be an independent risk factor for cardiovascular disease, acting through yet unidentified mechanisms (Hubert et al. 1982). Recent evidence indicates that obesity increases cardiac work and is associated with a higher incidence of congestive heart failure (Messerli 1982).

The compounded effect of other risk factors – such as hypertriglyceridaemia, hyperuricaemia, hypercholesterolaemia, hyperinsulinaemia and low serum HDL-cholesterol – although less important, must also be considered in obesity-related cardiovascular risk. Indeed, less than 10% of obese subjects are entirely free of one or more risk factors, and these are mainly younger, less obese subjects (Berchtold 1981, Patel et al. 1980). The Ad Hoc Committee of the Build and Blood Pressure Study (1980) has reconfirmed previous findings that incremental weight gains increase the risk of cardiovascular death. There is, therefore, no doubt that obesity, both independently and in association with other risk factors such as hypertension, is a deadly disease.

Mechanisms of hypertension in obesity

The occurrence of two very common disorders, obesity and essential hypertension, might suggest that the finding of hypertension in obese subjects is merely coincidental. This probably is not entirely true, though the question is unresolved. Both epidemiological and metabolic evidence indicate that obesity itself can lead to hypertension. Whether a unique form of hypertension exists that could be labelled 'obesity hypertension' remains to be established. Certainly many metabolic and haemodynamic derangements associated with obesity could contribute to blood pressure elevations (Table 1). This report will focus on sodium balances and the sympathetic nervous system as likely sources of hypertension in obesity.

Sodium balance

Dahl and co-workers (1958) first suggested that, in the process of ingesting more calories, obese subjects also take in more salt. This observation, which was left unchallenged for many years, was based on a study of a small number of obese hypertensive women for whom a low-calorie intake without concomitant salt restriction failed to lower blood pressure. Salt restriction alone or in combination with a hypocaloric diet lowered blood pressure in this study. Recent ovservations have cast doubt on the validity of some of these conclusions.

In a study of 81 obese hypertensive subjects in Israel, Reisen and co-workers (1978) put individuals on a low-calorie diet but specifically instructed them to eat generous servings of salty, low-calorie foods. Blood pressure reductions were quite striking (mean values: 26 mm Hg systolic, 20 mm Hg diastolic) and correlated well with the loss of body weight and occurred independent of salt intake during a two-month weight-loss period. In a second group of obese hypertensives, who were kept on antihypertensive medication, reductions in blood pressure during a high-salt, low-calorie diet were also striking. In an extension of this original report, Eliahou et al. (1981) studied 212 obese, hypertensive subjects on a balanced hypocaloric diet who were advised to eat salt freely. They noted that two thirds of compliant subjects achieved normal blood pres-

Table 1. Metabolic and haemodynamic abnormalities in obese subjects that could contribute to arterial hypertension

1. Increased cardiac output	5. Decreased Na^+, K^+ATPase pump activity
2. Increased vascular volume	6. Increased plasma renin activity
3. Increased sodium intake and excretion	7. Increased plasma aldosterone
4. Increased insulin levels	8. Increased plasma noradrenaline

sure levels with the loss of only one-half of their weight excess. Urinary sodium measurements showed that salt intake remained high, despite the drop in blood pressure that accompanied weight loss. It was concluded that, whatever role high sodium intake had in hypertension in obesity, its effect could be overridden by weight loss.

In a published report of 25 obese patients undergoing weight loss, 12 of whom had hypertension, we examined the influence of sodium intake on the hypotensive response to weight reduction by maintaining the subjects on high and low constant sodium intakes and carefully monitoring urinary sodium excretion (Tuck et al. 1981). During weight loss achieved by the supplemented fasting method (320 cal/day, 70 g protein, 50 g carbohydrate) the fall in blood pressure was identical in subjects during 12 weeks on 120 or 40 mEq sodium diets (Fig. 1). Compliance to the dietary sodium intake during the 12 weeks was documented by showing that urinary sodium excretion matched sodium intake. This study provided further proof that the potent hypotensive effect of weight reduction in the obese occurs independently of sodium balance. Pressures actually fell more rapidly in subjects receiving the higher sodium intake.

The renin-angiotensin system provides an important hormonal regulatory mechanism for maintaining blood pressure and might be expected to reflect abnormalities in sodium homoeostasis in obese subjects with hypertension. Correlations between levels of plasma renin activity and body weight have not been reported. Some studies have found normal ambient levels of plasma renin activity in obese subjects after standardizing for salt intake, age and other factors that effect this measurement (Mujais

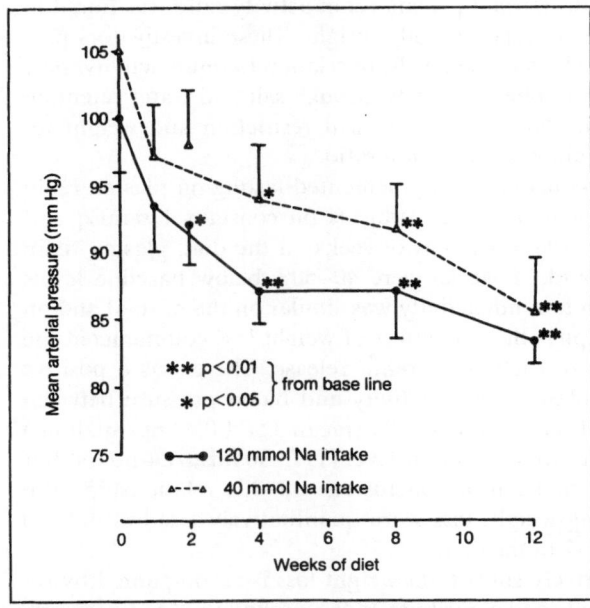

Fig. 1. Decrements in mean arterial pressure (mean ± SEM) during supplemented fasting in obese patients on a constant sodium intake (From Tuck et al. 1981, courtesy of the publishers, N Engl J Med).

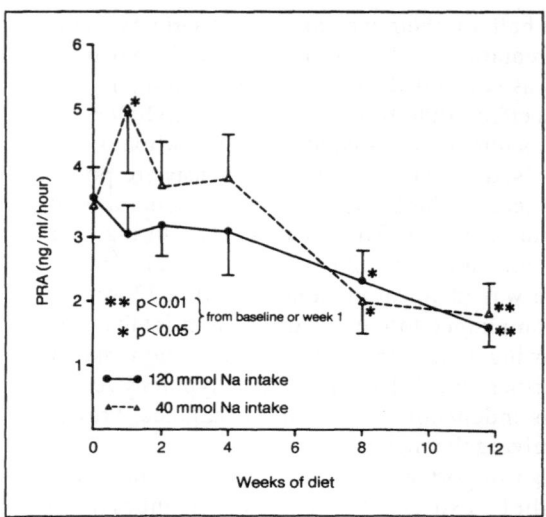

Fig. 2. Changes in plasma renin activity (PRA, mean ± SEM) during weight loss by supplemented fasting in obese patients (From Tuck et al. 1981, courtesy of the publishers, N Engl J Med).

et al. 1982; Messerli 1982; Boehringer et al. 1982). One investigation found relatively low levels of renin but normal aldosterone values in obese hypertensive subjects (Hiramatsu et al. 1981). The aldosterone: plasma renin activity ratio was found to increase progressively with increases in relative body weight. These investigators proposed that the inappropriately high aldosterone levels, in relation to renin activity, play a role in the genesis of hypertension in obese subjects through salt and water retention and volume expansion. Thiazide diuretics, as well as salt restriction and weight reduction, reversed the inappropriate aldosterone: renin ratio.

We examined the effect of weight reduction by supplemented fasting on plasma renin activity and aldosterone concentrations in obese subjects on constant 120 mEq and 40 mEq sodium intakes (Tuck et al. 1981). After two weeks on the diet, plasma renin levels started to decline and at 8 and 12 weeks were 40–50% below baseline levels (Fig. 2). The magnitude of reduction in renin activity was similar on the normal and on the sodium-restricted diets. This implies that the effect of weight loss counteracted the usual stimulatory effect of sodium restriction on renin release. There was a positive correlation between reductions in plasma renin activity and blood pressure between weeks 4 and 12. Baseline levels of plasma renin activity (mean 3.56±0.42 ng/ml/hour) were high when related to the mean urinary sodium level (197±30 mEq/24-hours) but the study group was too small to make firm conclusions on this relationship. The changes in aldosterone levels during weight loss were quantitatively less but did fall significantly from baseline by week 12 of the diet.

These results demonstrate that relatively short-term weight loss is accompanied by reductions in plasma renin activity that may contribute to the decline in blood pressure. Whether similar changes in renin and aldosterone occur with more prolonged, less calorie-restricted diets is uncertain. Reisin et al. (1983) studied 12 obese, hypertensive sub-

100

jects for an average of nine months of weight loss with a balanced hypocaloric diet. They reported that plasma noradrenaline levels fell significantly but plasma renin activity did not. It also appears that the pressor response to infusion of angiotensin II in mild-to-moderately obese hypertensives is similar to that in normal weight hypertensive subjects (Boehringer et al. 1982). These investigators concluded that there was no unique aberration in the renin-angiotensin system and in the cardiovascular responses to angiotensin II in overweight compared to lean hypertensive subjects.

These studies do not, however, exclude the possibility that more basic mechanisms in sodium homoeostasis and transport are important factors in the hypertension of obesity. Obese subjects and animals have reduced activity of the Na^+ transport pump system (Na^+, K^+ dependent ATPase pump) in certain cells (York et al. 1978; Lin et al. 1978; Sowers et al. 1982 b). Although this factor could be important in the development of hypertension, we have recently reported very little change in erythrocyte Na^+, K^+ATPase activity in obese patients during the decline in blood pressure which accompanies reductions in body weight (Sowers et al. 1982 b).

Sympathetic nervous system

An adaptive response of the sympathetic nervous system to changes in nutrient availability is known to exist and has certain survival value, especially in times of famine. Contrary to the belief that calorific excess diminishes sympathetic nervous system activity, excess caloric intake appears to stimulate it. A more precise definition of this relationship is hampered by limitations in the methods for measuring the activity of the sympathetic nervous system in man. Measurement of urinary or circulating levels of catecholamines offers the only practical method, but the complex disposal of these compounds means that this method should only be viewed as a partial measurement of sympathetic nervous activity.

The effect of fasting and sucrose feeding on cardiac noradrenaline turnover in rats was first reported by Young and Landsberg (1977; 1979). In comparison with controls, the calculated noradrenaline turnover rate was decreased by 39% in fasted rats and increased by 129% in sucrose-overfed rats. Thus, fasting suppressed and overfeeding stimulated sympathetic nervous system outflow. These adaptations appear to occur rapidly, within one or two days of the start of the diet, and persist as long as the diet is maintained. The nature of the caloric signal to the regulation of the sympathetic nervous system has also been elucidated. Although both carbohydrate and protein overfeeding stimulate sympathetic activity, the response to protein is delayed, which suggests that the conversion of protein to glucose is a necessary first step. The importance of carbohydrate in this response suggests that the insulin response to glucose could participate in altering sympathetic activity.

Excess energy intake through induction of increased sympathetic nervous system outflow could result in an increase in blood pressure. A major function of the sympathoadrenal system is regulation of blood pressure. It would therefore seem reasonable to expect energy excess to have an effect on blood pressure through stimulation of this system. In the spontaneously hypertensive rat, caloric restriction lowers blood pressure (Young et al. 1978). The hypocaloric diet reduced blood pressure by 14% and overfeeding with sucrose produced a significant 10% increment in blood pressure.

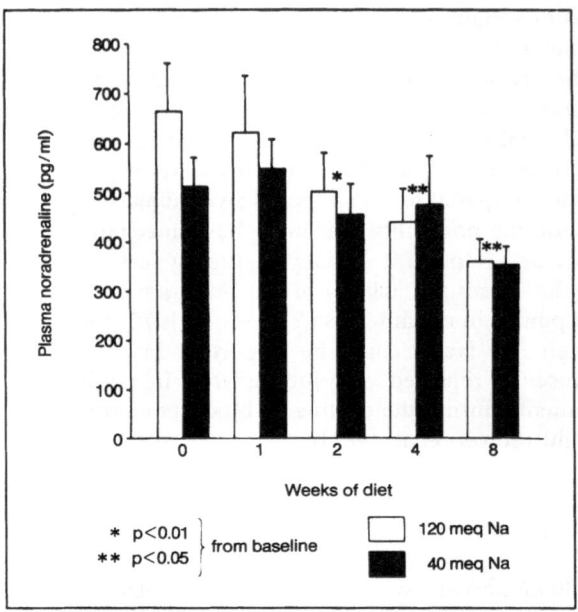

Fig. 3. Changes in plasma noradrenaline responses (mean ± SEM) to upright posture (10 minutes) during 8 weeks of supplemented fasting on two sodium intakes (From Tuck et al., 1983, courtesy of the publishers, Acta Endocrinologica).

These studies imply that in this animal model there is an influence of diet on the maintenance of blood pressure. We do not know whether this is also the case in man, but one could imagine a situation in which carbohydrate assimilation would stimulate sympathetic activity and increase arterial pressure.

Sympathetic nervous system activity appears to be increased in obese subjects (Jung et al. 1980; Sowers et al. 1982 a). The patients in our own study (Tuck et al. 1983), who were more than 25% over ideal body weight, showed both supine and upright plasma noradrenaline levels approximately 30% greater than values in matched non-obese subjects (Fig. 3). Mean ambulatory levels of plasma noradrenaline ranged from 420 to 1440 pg/ml in obese subjects; these values are high enough to produce adrenergic-mediated changes in cardiovascular function. Subsequently, obese subjects were placed on a supplemented fasting programme, at two different levels of sodium intake, and blood pressure, body weight and plasma noradrenaline levels were monitored at intervals of 1–2 weeks for eight weeks. Weight reduction by supplemented fasting was accompanied by significant reductions in blood pressure. Both these events were directly correlated with significant, step-wise reductions in ambient plasma noradrenaline levels (Fig. 3). These changes started approximately two weeks after starting the low-calorie diet; after 8 weeks, plasma noradrenaline concentration had fallen to the same levels as in non-obese controls. The decline in blood pressure and noradrenaline often occurred before obese subjects had reached ideal body weight. These observations suggest that the reductions in blood pressure that occur during weight reduction are secondary to reductions in plasma noradrenaline levels, which are in turn a function of reduced sympathetic nervous system activity.

Whether the high ambient plasma noradrenaline levels in obesity hypertension relate to changes in metabolism or in vascular sensitivity is not known. A study of noradrenaline infusion in overweight normotensive and essential hypertensive subjects has shown that pressor sensitivity to noradrenaline infusion and noradrenaline clearance are both normal (Boehringer et al. 1982). Another study has compared changes in vascular volume and systemic and regional haemodynamics with changes in plasma noradrenaline before and after weight reduction (Reisin et al. 1983). Total volume of circulating and cardiopulmonary blood were reduced after weight reduction, which resulted in decreases in cardiac output and arterial blood pressure, accompanied by a significant decline in concentrations of resting mean plasma noradrenaline from 591 ± 22 ng/l to 261 ± 51 ng/l. These data suggest that reduced adrenergic activity could contribute to the redistribution of intravascular blood away from the cardiopulmonary area, which would reduce venous return, cardiac output and arterial pressure. Thus, it may be feasible in the future to propose a major role for the sympathetic nervous system in the genesis of arterial hypertension in obesity. The high levels of circulating noradrenaline may also explain certain associated findings in obesity, including the increased values of plasma renin activity, increased cardiac output, increased sodium reabsorption and other factors that could be secondary to increased sympathetic activity.

Treatment of obese subjects with hypertension

Guidelines for the control of blood pressure in obese hypertensive subjects, both with and without drugs, are generally lacking. Several large-scale clinical trials have demonstrated that mortality is reduced when intervention drug therapy is used to lower blood pressure in essential hypertensives (Veterans Administration Cooperative Study Group on Antihypertensive Agents 1967, 1970 and 1977). Unfortunately, obesity was not adequately considered in these trials, though it must be presumed that a certain number of subjects with essential hypertension would be over ideal body weight. Several studies have documented the beneficial effects of weight reduction on lowering blood pressure. However, with a few exceptions, such as the Evans Country study (Tyroler et al. 1975), few of these studies involved large-scale community trials with long-term efforts at both weight reduction and maintenance of weight loss. In addition, almost nothing is known about the comparative merits of controlling hypertension in obesity with or without drugs. For example, we know very little about the effect of obesity on the metabolism, side-effects and efficacy of routine antihypertensive agents.

Weight reduction

Many clinical trials have now established that weight reduction is accompanied by very significant reductions in arterial blood pressure (Tyroler et al. 1975; Berchtold et al.

1982; Tuck et al. 1981 and 1983; Sowers et al. 1982 a; Chiang et al. 1969; Ramsay et al. 1978; Fletcher 1954). Weight reduction appears to have a greater hypotensive effect than sodium restriction. In fact, obesity may be more directly related to hypertension than sodium intake (Dustan 1983).

Several investigations have attempted to examine the rate of blood pressure reduction associated with a given weight loss. The Multiple Risk Factors Intervention Trial (1976), for example, noted that for each 1.8 kg fall in body weight there was a 1 mm Hg reduction in diastolic pressure. In another study of obese females, a loss of 6.4 kg yielded a 30 mm Hg fall in systolic pressure and 19 mm Hg in disatolic pressure (Fletcher 1954). Reisen et al. (1980) in a study from Israel reported a marked fall in blood pressure in obese hypertensives with moderate weight loss. Patients who lost about 9.5 kg displayed a mean reduction in systolic pressure of 26 mm Hg and diastolic 20 mm Hg.

Another interesting feature of weight reduction is that even in normotensive subjects it yields some reduction of blood pressure. Indeed, blood pressure often 'normalizes' before ideal body weight is attained. Some observers have found that a weight loss as low as 5–10% is sufficient to significantly lower or normalize blood pressure in certain obese hypertensive persons. This is an important finding, since many doctors are sceptical about the place of long-term weight control in the management of hypertension. It needs to be re-emphasized that obese subjects do not need to attain ideal body weight to effect significant falls in blood pressure. This has been confirmed in such large trials as the Multiple Risk Factor Intervention Trial (MRFIT; 1976), the Chicago Coronary Prevention Evaluation Program (Stamler et al. 1978) and the Evans County, Georgia study (Tyroler et al. 1975). In the MRFIT programme a loss in weight of 5% or more substantially reduced the risk of coronary heart disease, which presumably would have correlated with a reduction in blood pressure. As emphasized by Sims (1982), the 'stepped-care' approach to the treatment of hypertensives who are obese needs to be revised so that the initial steps in blood pressure control include characterization of a number of factors, including metabolic derangements, reduction of energy intake, increased physical activity, education and long-term behavioural maintenance support. Suprisingly small changes in the lifestyle of the sedentary, overeating, underexercising, obese hypertensive may yield remarkable results. Recent experience with very-low-calorie diet programmes suggests that a larger trial of this approach to obese hypertensives should be considered (Tuck et al. 1981; Tuck et al. 1983; Sowers et al. 1982 a), particularly in the moderate-to-massively-obese patient. For the less obese subject, who is perhaps 20% over ideal body weight, a balanced hypocaloric diet may suffice.

Antihypertensive therapy

Almost no clinical studies have specifically studied the use of antihypertensive agents in obese patients with hypertension. There are, however, some theoretical reasons for believing that obese hypertensives may differ from their lean hypertensive counterparts in the side-effects, adverse reactions and efficacy of these agents. It is also possible that some of the specific haemodynamic and hormonal abnormalities described in obese subjects, such as high cardiac output and increased sympathetic nervous system activity, may make certain antihypertensive agents more effective as a result of their mechanism of action. This concept of monotherapy, aimed at the correction of a specific abnormality in blood pressure control, is theoretically appealing and has only been partially realized in the treatment of essential hypertension.

Diuretic therapy should theoretically be particularly effective in obesity hypertension, since obese subjects are likely to take in more salt, which increases intravascular volume. However, this proposal has never been adequately tested; it would require a comparison of the efficacy of diuretics in treating lean and obese hypertensives. Our experience suggests that this would show a negative result, since only 15–20% of obese hypertensives normalize their blood pressure on diuretic therapy alone. This response rate is equal to that seen in non-obese hypertensives.

A further problem with diuretic agents is that they might accentuate metabolic derangements, including glucose intolerance, hyperuricaemia and hyperlipidaemia in obese hypertensives. Obesity itself is associated with an increased incidence of glucose intolerance, hypertriglyceridaemia, hypercholesterolaemia and hyperuricaemia. Thiazide diuretics could only increase these conditions in obese subjects, and it is therefore necessary to weigh the potential of these agents to lower blood pressure in obese hypertensives against these independent metabolic risk factors.

Vasodilator agents may also have only limited applicability in the treatment of the obese hypertensive. The haemodynamic characteristics of obesity hypertension, including increased cardiac output with less pronounced changes in peripheral vascular resistance, makes vasodilator therapy less suitable for this population. Since vasodilators increase heart rate and cardiac work, it might not be appropriate to use them alone in these subjects. Their effect on sodium retention would also seem inappropriate in a population which is known to have an increased intravascular volume. Thus, the use of vasodilators to treat obese hypertensives would require the addition of sympathetic inhibitors to attenuate their cardiovascular effects and diuretics to offset sodium retention. This amounts to triple drug therapy in a population which should not need it, since hypertension is usually only mild to moderate.

There are theoretical reasons for considering beta-adrenergic blocking agents for the treatment of obese hypertensives, mainly based on their ability to decrease cardiac output. It is uncertain whether this observation has ever been tested in clinical trials to compare the effect of beta-blockers in lean and obese hypertensive subjects. There is some evidence to the contrary, that beta-blockers may be less effective in obese hypertensive subjects especially with advancing age. Unfortunately none of these observations are well founded. Since long-term beta-blocking therapy may be associated with glucose intolerance and hyperlipidaemia, these factors should be closely monitored in the treatment of obese hypertensives.

Since high levels of circulating catecholamines are found in obese hypertensives, methods which reduce them may be the treatment of choice for individuals unable to lose weight. It is conceivable that high concentrations of noradrenaline stimulate renin secretion, affect cardiac output and, most importantly, increase peripheral resistance. However, few anti-hypertensive agents lead to reduced levels of circulating catecholamines. In fact, several agents, such as diuretics, vasodilators and beta-adrenergic agents, are associated with increases in plasma catecholamines.

The antihypertensive agent clonidine produces a significant reduction in circulating noradrenaline during chronic therapy. This may account for part of its antihypertensive action, although other mechanisms are also important. Preliminary evidence in our clinics suggests that clonidine monotherapy in obese hypertensives results in normalization of plasma noradrenaline levels and this correlates with control of blood pressure. Administration of clonidine as a single night-time dose minimizes the side-effects of sedation and dry mouth. As clonidine does not significantly alter glucose tolerance, does not increase cardiac output or cause major sodium retention, it may be well suited for therapy of obese hypertensive subjects where adequate weight loss is not attainable or cannot be sustained. During weight reduction therapy in a patient with significant hypertension, I would recommend antihypertensive control of blood pressure, since dietary trials are often prolonged and are not very successful on a large scale. Not treating high blood pressure during this period could place these individuals at increased risk. If weight reduction is successful, the antihypertensive therapy can be appropriately adjusted or withdrawn.

References

1 Ad Hoc Committee of the New Build and Blood Pressure Study, Build Study (1979). Chicago: Society of Actuaries and Association of Life Insurance Medical Directors of America.
2 Ashley FW Jr, Kannel WB (1974) Relation of weight change to changes in atherogenic traits: The Framingham Study. J Chronic Dis 27: 103–114.
3 Berchtold P, Berger M, Jörgens V, et al (1981) Cardiovascular risk factors and HDL-cholesterol levels in obesity. Int J Obes 5: 1–10.
4 Berchtold P, Jörgens V, Kemmer FW, Berger M (1982) Obesity and hypertension: cardiovascular response to weight reduction. Hypertension 4 (Suppl 3): III 50–III 55.
5 Berglund G, Ljungman S, Hartford M, Wilhelmsen L, Björntorp P (1982) Type of obesity and blood pressure. Hypertension 4: 692–696.
6 Boehringer K, Beretta-Piccoli C, Weidmann P, Meier A, Ziegler W (1982) Pressor factors and cardiovascular pressor responsiveness in lean and overweight normal and hypertensive subjects. Hypertension 4: 687–702.
7 Chiang BN, Perlman LV, Epstein FH (1969) Overweight and hypertension: A review. Circulation 39: 403–421.
8 Dahl LK, Silver L, Christie RW (1958) Role of salt in the fall of blood pressure accompanying reduction in obesity. N Engl J Med 258: 1186–1188.
9 Dahl LK (1972) Salt and hypertension. Am J Clin Nutr 25: 231–244.
10 DeLuise M, Blackburn GL, Flier JS (1980) Reduced activity of the red-cell sodium potassium pump in human obesity. N Engl J Med 303: 1017–1022.
11 Dustan HP (1983) Mechanisms of hypertension associated with obesity. Ann Intern Med 98 (Part 2): 860–864.
12 Eliahou HE, Iaina A, Gaon T, Shochat J, Modan M (1981) Body weight reduction necessary to attain normotension in the overweight hypertensive patient. Int J Obes 5 suppl 1: 157–163.
13 Fletcher AP (1954) The effect of weight reduction upon the blood pressure of obese hypertensive women. Q J Med 47: 331–345.
14 Gillum RF, Taylor HL, Brozek J, Polansky P, Blackburn M (1982) Indices of obesity and blood pressure in young men followed 32 years. J Chronic Dis 35: 211–219.
15 Gordon T, Kannel WB (1976) Obesity and cardiovascular disease: The Framingham Study. J Clin Endocrinol Metab 5: 367–375.
16 Harlan WR, Oberman A, Mitchell RE, Graybiel A (1973) A 30-year study of blood pressure in a white male cohort. In: Onesti G, Kim KE, Moyer JH (eds.) Hypertension: Mechanism and Management. Grune & Stratton: New York: 85–91.
17 Havlik RJ, Hubert HB, Fabsitz RR, Feinleib M (1983) Weight and hypertension. Ann Intern Med 98: 855–859.
18 Hiramatsu K, Yamada T, Ichikawa K, Izumiyama T, Nagata H (1981) Changes in endocrine activities relative to obesity in patients with essential hypertension. J Am Geriatr Soc 29: 25–30.
19 Hubert HB, Feinleib M, McNamara PM, Castelli WP (1982) Obesity as an independent risk factor for cardiovascular disease in Framingham (Abstract). CVD Epidemiol Newslett 31: 39.

20 Hypertensive Detection and Follow-up Program Cooperative Group: Five-year findings of the Hypertension Detection and Follow-up Program; reduction in mortality of persons with high blood pressure including mild hypertension. (1979) JAMA 242:2562–2571.

21 Jung RT, Shetty PS, James WPT (1980) Nutritional effects on thyroid catecholamine metabolism. Clin Sci 58:183–191.

22 Kannel WB, Brand N, Skinner JJ, Dawber TR, McNamara PN (1967) The relation of adiposity to blood pressure and development of hypertension: The Framingham Study. Anr Int Med 67:48–59.

23 Kannel WB, Gordon T (1968) Correlations. In: Kannel WB, Gordon T (eds.) The Framingham Study: An Epidemiological Investigation of Cardiovascular Disease. Washington DC: DHEW.

24 Lin MH, Romsos DR, Akera T, Leveille GA (1978) Na+-K+-ATPase enzyme units in skeletal muscle from lean and obese mice. Biochem Biophys Res Commun 80:398–404.

25 Lynds BG, Seyler SK, Morgan BM (1980) The relationship between elevated blood pressure and obesity in black children. Am J Public Health 70:171–173.

26 Maxwell MH, Waks AU, Schroth PC, Karam M, Dornfeld LP (1982) Error in blood pressure measurement due to incorrect cuff size in obese patients. Lancet ii:33–36.

27 McCue CM, Miller WW, Mauck HP, Robertson L, Parr EL (1979) Adolescent blood pressure in Richmond, Virginia, schools. Virginia Med 106:210–220.

28 Messerli FH (1982) Cardiovascular effects of obesity and hypertension. Lancet i:1165–1168.

29 Mujais SK, Tarazi RC, Dustan HP, Fouad RM, Bravo EL (1982) Hypertension in obese patients: haemodynamic and volume studies. Hypertension 4:84–92.

30 Multiple Risk Factor Intervention Trial Research Group: The multiple risk factor intervention trial (MRFIT); A national study of primary prevention of heart disease. (1976) JAMA 235; 825–828.

31 Patel YC, Eggen DA, Strong JP (1980) Obesity, smoking and atherosclerosis: a study of interassociations. Atherosclerosis 36:481–490.

32 Ramsay LE, Ramsay MH, Hettiarachchi J, Davies DL, Winchester J (1978) Weight reduction in a blood pressure clinic. Br Med J 2:244–245.

33 Reisin E, Frohlich ED, Messerli FH, Dreslinski GR, Dunn FG, Jones MM, Batson HM (1983) Cardiovascular changes after weight reduction in obesity hypertension. Ann Int Med 98:315–319.

34 Reisin E, Abel R, Modan M, Silverberg DS, Eliahou HE, Modan B (1978) Effect of weight loss without salt restriction on the reduction of blood pressure in overweight hypertensive patients. N Engl J Med 298:1–6.

35 Schacter J, Kuller LH, Perfetti C (1982) Blood pressure during the first two years of life. Am J Epidemiol 116:29–41.

36 Siervogel RM, Roche AF, Chumlea WC, Morris JG, Webb P, Knittle JL (1982) Blood pressure, body composition, and fat tissue cellularity in adults. Hypertension 4:382–386.

37 Sims EAH (1982) Mechanisms of hypertension in the overweight. Hypertension 4 (suppl 3): III 43–III 49.

38 Sowers JR, Whitfield LA, Catania RA, Stern N, Tuck ML, Dornfeld L, Maxwell M (1982a) Role of the sympathetic nervous system in blood pressure maintenance in obesity. J Clin Endocrinol Metab 54:1181–1185.

39 Sowers JR, Whitfield L, Beck FWJ, et al (1982b) Role of enhanced sympathetic nervous system activity and reduced Na+-K+-dependent adenosine triphosphatase activity in maintenance of elevated blood pressure in obesity: effects of weight loss. Clin Sci 63:121s–124s.

40 Stamler R, Stamler J, Riedlinger WF, Algera G, Roberts RM (1978) Weight and blood pressure: findings in hypertension screening of 1 million Americans. JAMA 240:1607–1610.

41 Tuck ML, Sowers J, Dornfeld L, Kledzick G, Maxwell M (1981) The effect of weight reduction on blood pressure, plasma renin activity, and plasma aldosterone levels in obese patients. N Engl J Med 304:930–933.

42 Tuck ML, Sowers JR, Dornfeld L, Whitfield L, Maxwell M (1983) Reductions in plasma catecholamines and blood pressure during weight loss in obese subjects. Acta Endocrinol 102:252–257.

43 Tyroler HA, Heyden S, Hames CG (1975) Weight and hypertension: Evans County studies of blacks and whites. In Paul O (ed.) Epidemiology and Control of Hypertension. Stratton Intercontinental: New York: 177–201.

44 York DA, Bray GA, Yukimura Y (1978) An enzymatic defect in the obese (ob/ob) mouse: Loss of thyroid-induced sodium- and potassium-dependent adenosine triphosphatase. Proc Natl Acad Sci, USA 75:477–481.
45 Young JB, Landsberg L (1977) Suppression of sympathetic nevous system during fasting. Science 196:1473–1475.
46 Young JB, Landsberg L (1979) Effect of diet and cold exposure on norepinephrine turnover in pancreas and liver. Am J Physiol 236:E524–E533.
47 Young JB, Mullen D, Landsberg L (1978) Caloric restriction lowers blood pressure in the spontaneously hypertensive rat. Metabolism 27:1711–1714.
48 Veterans Administration Cooperative Study Group on Antihypertensive Agents: Effect of treatment on morbidity in hypertension; Results of patients with diastolic blood pressure averaging 115–129 (1967) JAMA 202:116–122.
49 Veterans Administration Cooperative Study Group on Antihypertensive Agents: Effects of treatment on morbidity in hypertension II. Results in patients with diastolic blood pressure averaging 90 through 114 mm Hg. (1970) JAMA 213:1143–1152.
50 Veterans Administration Cooperative Study on Antihypertensive Agents: Propranolol in the treatment of essential hypertension (1977) JAMA 237:2303–2310.

Correspondence:
Michael Tuck, M.D.
Chief of Endocrinology and Metabolism
VA Medical Center
16111 Plummer St.
Sepulveda, CA 91343

Discussion

HAYDUK:
Do you think that obese people need larger doses of antihypertensive drugs?

TUCK:
My impression is that they have not needed larger doses. In fact, if anything the contrary is true. However, we treated a group with relatively mild hypertension. Perhaps the one exception is beta-blocker treatment; here I think obese people might require bigger doses.

PEART:
With the obese patients you're dealing with, are you worried about the forearm circumference when you're measuring the blood pressure?

TUCK:
We measured the forearm circumference in each patient and used a series of blood pressure cuff sizes. I don't think, in this study, there need be concern about the falseness of the readings.

POLINSKY:
I would like to highlight some of the things that you said with respect to correlating weight and sympathetic drive. Some studies of anorexia nervosa support what you've been saying. It has been shown that the sympathetic nervous system in these patients has really toned down, and when we feed them we may actually turn the sympathetic nervous system back on. This may be the other end of the story you have discussed, namely that obesity is associated with increased sympathetic activity.

TUCK:
I think that's been pretty well documented.

Clonidine for treating patients with mild hypertension and angina pectoris

T. Zaleska, L. Ceremużyński

Introduction

An increase in the activity of the adrenergic nervous system is one of the features of mild hypertension and is thought to contribute to the mechanism of the disease (De Quatro and Chan 1972; Champlain et al. 1981). Both hypertension and augmented sympathetic drive help to produce the symptoms of angina pectoris by increasing afterload and accelerating metabolic rate, respectively. Each of these mechanisms raises the oxygen demand of the heart muscle and is likely to lead to a shortage of oxygen, which is known to trigger coronary pain.

It is well known that treatment plans for angina should, if necessary, include measures for normalizing blood pressure. The most suitable drug for this purpose is therefore one which has some action on the adrenergic nervous system.

Clonidine, an imidazoline derivative, is a drug which acts on the central nervous system and produces a decrease in sympathetic outflow from the brain (Kobinger and Walland 1967; Schmitt et al. 1967). Hence, it is likely to be useful for treating patients with both hypertension and angina pectoris, who are numerous in everyday clinical practice. To test this assumption we administered clonidine to a group of patients with mild hypertension and concomitant frequent coronary pains, for whom routine therapy was ineffective.

Subjects

During a period of 4 years starting on 20 January 1978, 92 patients were referred to the out-patient department of our clinic suffering from chronic angina resistant to routine medical therapy, such as long-acting nitrates, beta-blockers and calcium antagonists. They reported at least five coronary pains a week and displayed typical ischaemic features on an ECG.

Thirty-one of the patients also had mild hypertension within the range 170/90–200/110 mm Hg, and had been previously treated with hypotensive agents – thiazides and beta-blockers. Although their blood pressure was controlled for short periods of time, the symptoms of angina persisted. These 31 patients were considered to be suitable for the study group.

During a 2-week run-in period the patients kept a daily record of the number of coronary pains they had and their consumption of glyceryl trinitrate tablets. Intake of routine drugs (beta-blockers and long-acting nitrates) remained unchanged.

Twenty-five of the patients did not improve and displayed at least five coronary pains a week and an increased blood pressure within the range 160/90 mm Hg–190/

109

110 mm Hg. These 25 patients ultimately formed the study group. This group was made up of men and women free from other diseases with a mean age of 59.8 years (range 42–73 years). Myocardial infarction six months or more before the study was diagnosed in 12 cases.

Design of the study

This was a single-blind controlled trial. The clonidine and placebo tablets were identical in appearance and taste. During the trial, patients were reviewed weekly. Clonidine was given in a dose of 75 μg (one tablet) twice daily. Therapy lasted two weeks, either on placebo or on clonidine after a preliminary period on placebo. Routine coronary drugs used before the trial were maintained, except that beta-blockers were withdrawn before clonidine administration.

Biochemical methods

Free adrenaline (AD) and noradrenaline (NA) in a 24-hour sample of urine were determined fluorimetrically by the technique of Euler and Lishajko (1959) as modified by Górny (1964). The normal upper limits of AD and NA were 7.5 μg/24 hours and 37 μg/24 hours, respectively.

Efficacy evaluation

The number of episodes of angina and the consumption of glyceryl trinitrate tablets served as indices of clinical progress. The patients were considered to have improved if the number of coronary pains decreased by at least 50%. The results were statistically analysed using the Finney test (Finney et al. 1963).

Results

The results obtained in patients treated either with clonidine or placebo are shown in Table 1. Clonidine administration resulted in significant decrease in coronary pain ($p < 0.005$) and a reduction in the number of glyceryl trinitrate tablets consumed ($p < 0.05$). Blood pressure, both systolic and diastolic, decreased significantly on clonidine ($p < 0.005$) and the value of the double product (blood pressure × heart rate) was also considerably diminished ($p < 0.01$). Heart rate did not change. Urinary excretion of AD and NA decreased significantly in patients on clonidine ($p < 0.05$ and $p < 0.025$, respectively).

Figures 1–8 show the results of clonidine treatment in individual patients. Figure 1 shows the incidence of coronary pains. Twelve patients improved on clonidine, i.e. the number of their coronary pains decreased by at least 50% ($p < 0.005$). Another 13 cases did not meet this criterion although some of them displayed fewer coronary pains.

As shown in Fig. 2, the consumption of glyceryl trinitrate decreased in all but one of those patients who displayed clinical improvement ($p < 0.01$) and was slightly lowered in most of those who did not improve significantly.

Table 1. Comparison of clonidine and placebo in the treatment of patients with angina and mild hypertension (mean values for all patients, n = 25)

Regimen	Coronary pains (no. per week)	Glyceryl trinitrate tablets (no. per week)	Systolic blood pressure (mm Hg)	Diastolic blood pressure (mm Hg)	Heart rate (beats per min)	Double product (blood pressure × beats per min)	Adrenaline in urine (µg/24 hours)	Noradrenaline in urine (µg/24 hours)
Placebo	17.1	8.3	167.8	96.8	77.6	13.079	9.3	34.3
Clonidine	11.6	4.45	148.6	85.6	71.5	10.669	7.25	30.9
Upper limit of probability level	0.005	0.05	0.005	0.005	ns	0.01	0.05	0.025

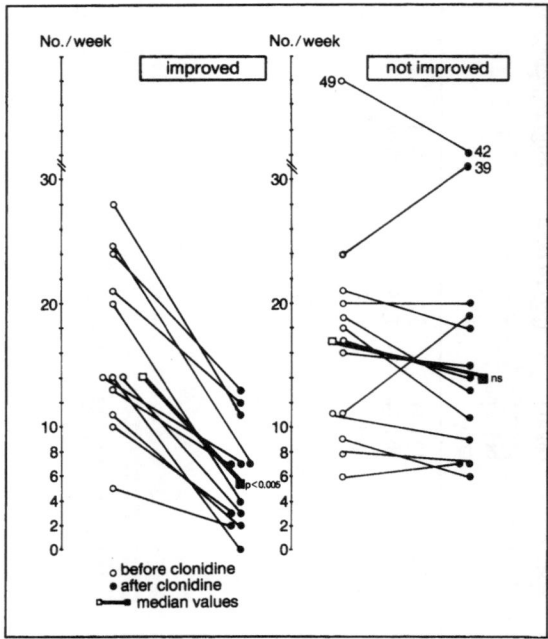

Fig. 1. The effect of clonidine upon the frequency of coronary pains in individual patients with angina and mild hypertension. Improved (patients with a decrease of at least 50%) n = 12; not improved n = 13

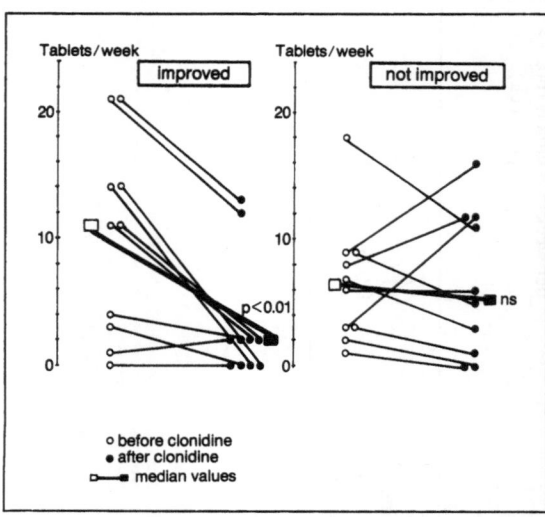

Fig. 2. The effect of clonidine upon the consumption of glyceryl trinitrate tablets in individual patients with angina and mild hypertension. Improved n = 10; not improved n = 10

112

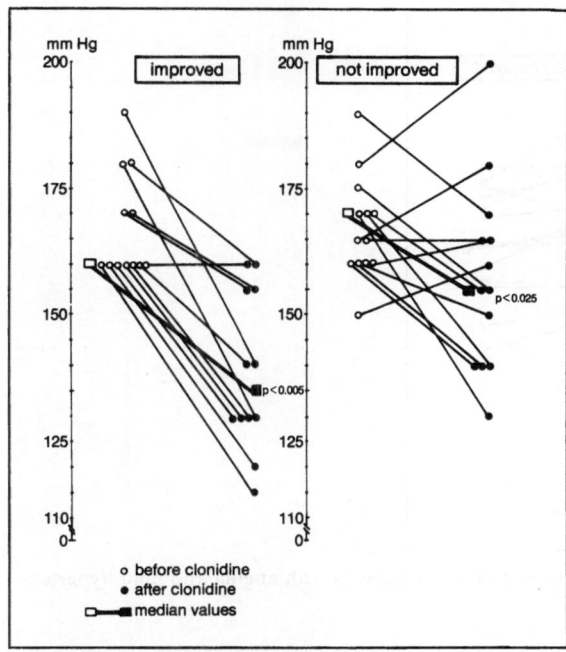

Fig. 3. The effect of clonidine upon systolic blood pressure in individual patients with angina and mild hypertension. Improved n = 12; not improved n = 13

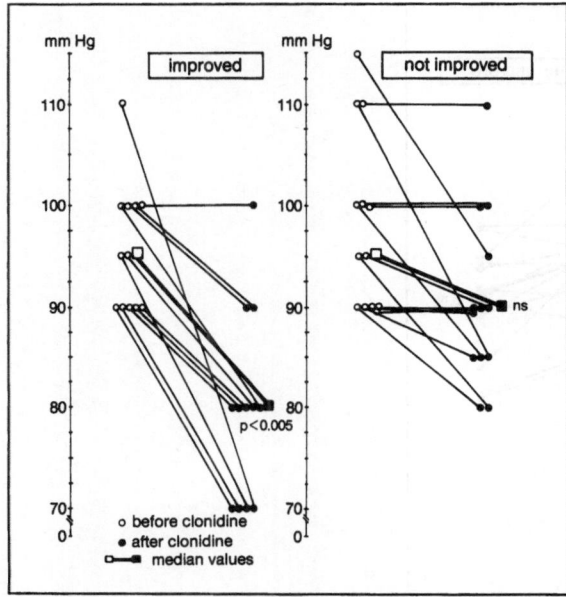

Fig. 4. The effect of clonidine upon diastolic blood pressure in individual patients with angina and mild hypertension. Improved n = 12; not improved n = 13

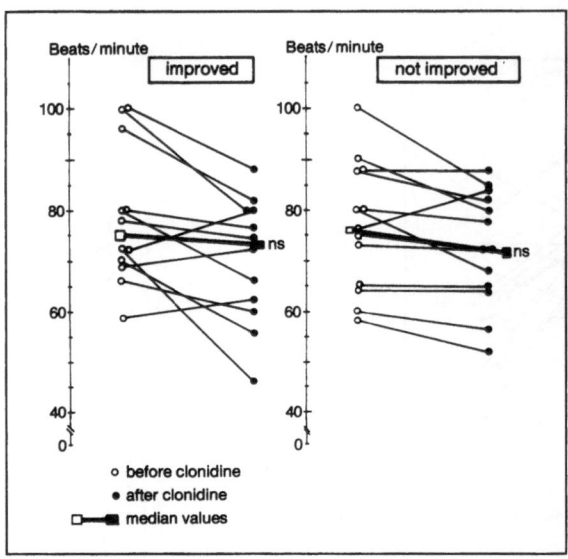

Fig. 5. The effect of clonidine on heart rate in individual patients with angina and mild hypertension. Improved n = 12; not improved n = 13.

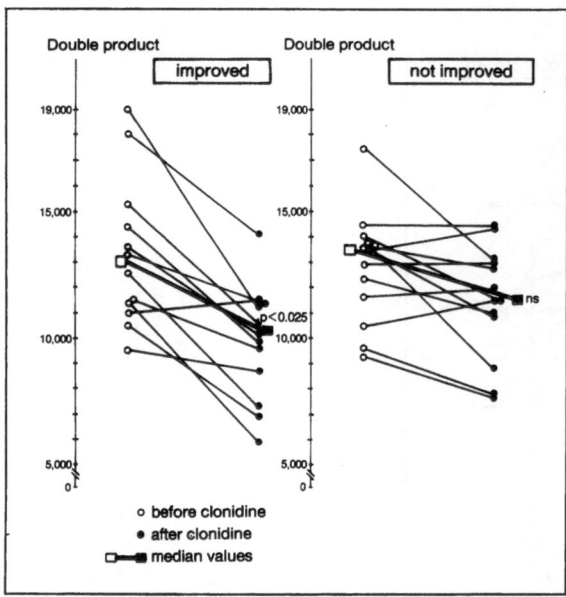

Fig. 6. The effect of clonidine on the value of the double product (blood pressure × heart rate) in individual patients with angina and mild hypertension. Improved n = 12; not improved n = 13.

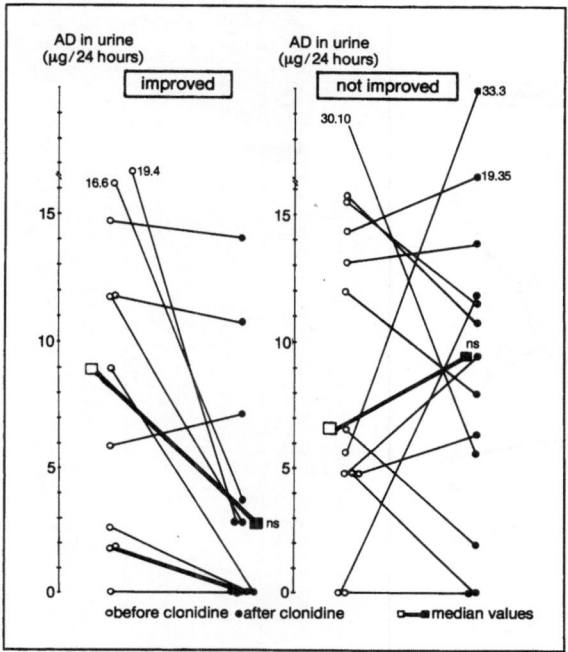

Fig. 7. The effect of clonidine upon urinary excretion of adrenaline in individual patients with angina and mild hypertension. Improved n = 11; not improved n = 13.

Clinical improvement on clonidine was accompanied by a significant decrease in both systolic (p < 0.005) and diastolic (p < 0.005) blood pressures, as shown in Figs 3 and 4.

Heart rate did not change significantly in either group of patients (Fig. 5), whereas the value of the double product considerably decreased in subjects who showed clinical improvement (p < 0.025; Fig. 6).

Changes in the excretion of both AD and NA after clonidine were not significantly related to clinical improvement (Figs 7 and 8). However, amongst the 11 patients who improved on clonidine, AD excretion decreased in nine cases and NA in seven cases. This tendency was not seen in patients who did not improve on clonidine therapy.

Discussion

This study has revealed that clonidine is an efficient drug in patients suffering from angina pectoris with concomitant mild hypertension.

It should be stressed that although coronary pains were resistant to routine therapy with long-lasting nitrates and beta-blockers, considerable improvement was achieved with clonidine in about half of the group. The drug regimen used was well tolerated and side-effects (dry mouth) were reported in only three patients, who nonetheless completed the trial.

At the dose prescribed, clonidine normalized blood pressure in the vast majority of patients, but not all these cases showed attenuation of angina. On the contrary, in some

115

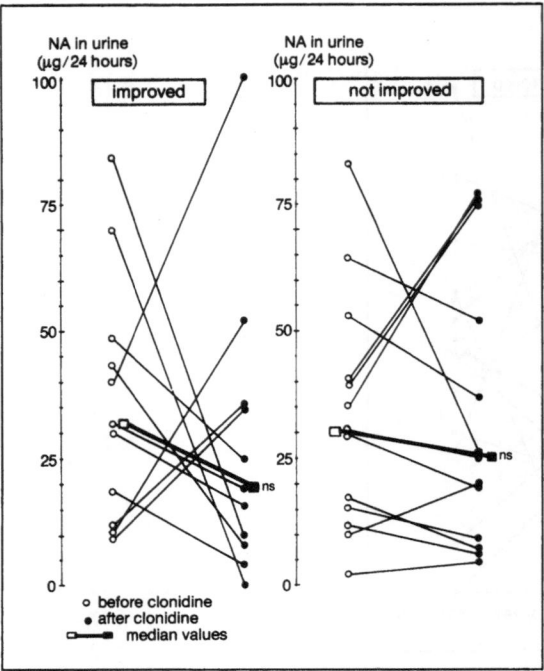

Fig. 8. The effect of clonidine upon urinary excretion of noradrenaline in individual patients with angina and mild hypertension. Improved n = 11; not improved n = 13.

subjects blood pressure remained high even though distinct clinical improvement was observed. The reason for this is that excessive cardiac work due to an increased afterload was responsible for angina in only a fraction of patients, which is in agreement with our earlier findings (Ceremużyński et al. 1979 a; Ceremużyński et al. 1979 b). In this study, we observed that clonidine was also effective in patients with normal blood pressure, which suggests that reduction of afterload is not its sole mechanism of operation. It is likely that the beneficial clinical effect of clonidine is also due to its reduction of adrenergic activity.

The level of activity of the sympathetic nervous systen can be monitored by measuring the daily excretion of urinary catecholamines. We have previously shown that clonidine decreases the excretion of AD and NA in healthy subjects (Ceremużyński et al. 1979 a) and in patients with angina (Ceremużyński et al. 1979 b). This was confirmed in the present study.

In several patients considerable reduction in of the excretion of AD and/or NA was observed, together with a decrease in the number of chest pains. Only in a few cases were catecholamine levels in urine reduced after clonidine, although the level of angina was still maintained (Figs 7 and 8).

Evidence exists to support a reciprocal relationship between the activity of the sympathetic nervous system and the clinical course of ischaemic heart disease (Raab 1963;

Mueller and Ayres 1978). High levels of catecholamines increase the demand of heart muscle for oxygen by augmenting the metabolic rate, and also by inducing an oxygen wasting effect (Challoner and Steinberg 1966). Thus the observed decrease in the level of excreted catecholamines found during clonidine therapy may be causally linked with the associated improvement in clinical symptoms.

Conclusions

Clonidine is a suitable drug for patients with angina and hypertension. It acts by reducing the activity of the sympathetic nervous system, which is a common aetiological factor in both ailments. Results obtained with the drug are very encouraging; it brought about clinical improvement in almost 50% of patients when added to routine regimens for treating angina and hypertension.

References

1 Ceremużyński L, Łada J, Maruchin M, Dłużniewski M, Herbaczyńska-Cedro K (1979 a) Suppression of catecholamine excretion by low doses of clonidine in healthy subjects and feasibility study on clonidine application in angina pectoris. Drug Res 5:829–835.
2 Ceremużyński L, Zaleska T, Łada W, Zalewski A (1979 b) Clonidine effect in chronic angina pectoris. Double-blind, crossover trial on 60 patients. Eur J Cardiol 10:415–427.
3 Challoner DR, Steinberg D (1966) Oxidative metabolism of myocardium as influenced by fatty acids and epinephrine. Am J Physiol 211:897–902.
4 Champlain J, Cousineau D, Lapointe L, Lavalee M, Nadean R, Denis G (1981) Sympathetic abnormalities in human hypertension. Clin Exp Hypertension 3:417–438.
5 De Quattro V, Chan S (1972) Raised plasma catecholamines in some patients with primary hypertension. Lancet i:806–809.
6 Finney DJ, Latscha R, Benett BM, Hsu P (1963) Tables for testing significance in a 2×2 contingency table. Cambridge University Press, Cambridge.
7 Górny D (1964) Fluorimetric determination of free adrenaline and noradrenaline in urine (in Polish). Pol Tyg Lek 19:632–635.
8 Kobinger W, Walland A (1967) Investigations into the mechanisms of the hypotensive effect of 2-(2,6-dichlorophenylamino)-2-imidazoline HCl. Eur J Pharmacol 2:155–162.
9 Mueller HS, Ayres SM (1978) Metabolic responses of the heart in acute myocardial infarction in man. Am J Cardiol 42:363–371.
10 Raab W (1963) The nonvascular metabolic myocardial vulnerability factor in "coronary heart disease". Am Heart J 66:685–706.
11 Schmitt H, Schmitt H, Boissier JR, Giudicelli JF (1967) Centrally mediated decrease in sympathetic tone induced by 2-(2,6-dichlorophenylamino)-2-imidazoline (ST 155, Catapresan). Eur J Pharmacol 2:147–148.
12 von Euler US, Lishajko F (1959) The estimation of catecholamines in urine. Acta Physiol Scand 45:122–132.

Correspondence:
Dr. L. Ceremużyński
Department of Cardiology, Postgraduate Medical School
Grochowski Hospital, Grenadierów 51/59
04007 Warsaw, Poland.

New pharmacological approaches in the treatment of mild hypertension. The potential role of converting enzyme inhibitors and calcium blocking agents

F. Alhenc-Gelas, P. Corvol, J. Menard

Control of blood pressure in hypertension has generally been achieved in the past by the use of diuretics and betablockers, either alone or in combination with vasodilators or drugs interacting with the sympathetic nervous system. These treatments obviously have highly beneficial effects since several controlled trials have shown that lowering of blood pressure reduces cardiovascular mortality and morbidity in treated hypertensive patients. (Australian Therapeutic Trial of Mild Hypertension 1980; Smith 1977; Veterans Administration Cooperative Study Group 1970). There are, however, some limitations in this approach to the treatment of hypertension. In approximately two thirds of unselected patients, satisfactory control of blood pressure is not obtained with the drug of first choice alone. Therefore it is often necessary to prescribe two or more drugs. The antihypertensive effect of diuretics can be limited by overstimulation of the renin-angiotensin system (Alhenc-Gelas et al. 1978; Laragh 1973) and that of vasodilators by sodium retention (Ibsen et al. 1978). Side-effects such as postural hypotension, disturbance of the microcirculation or erectile dysfunction are not uncommon (Smith 1977). Recently, two new classes of antihypertensive agent: converting enzyme inhibitors and calcium channel blockers, became available for the treatment of hypertension (Table 1). Although their mechanisms of action vary they are all able to decrease vascular resistance and lower blood pressure in patients with mild to severe hypertension.

Angiotensin converting enzyme (ACE) inhibitors

The design of ACE inhibitors is a result of a new and logical approach to the treatment of hypertension. Many antihypertensive drugs, including diuretics, betablockers and calcium antagonists, were not originally designed as antihypertensive agents but ACE inhibitors were specifically synthesized to act as inhibitors of the renin-angiotensin system. ACE inhibitors block the conversion of angiotensin I, produced by the action of renin on angiotensinogen, into the pressor peptide angiotensin II (Cushman et al. 1977). After oral or intravenous administration of an ACE inhibitor the increase in blood pressure induced by angiotensin I is reduced or abolished, whereas the pressor

Table 1. Antihypertensive therapy in the 80's – Expected improvements

1 Improvement in the health care distribution system
2 Better use of old drugs
3 Introduction of new drugs:
 • converting enzyme inhibitors
 • calcium antagonists

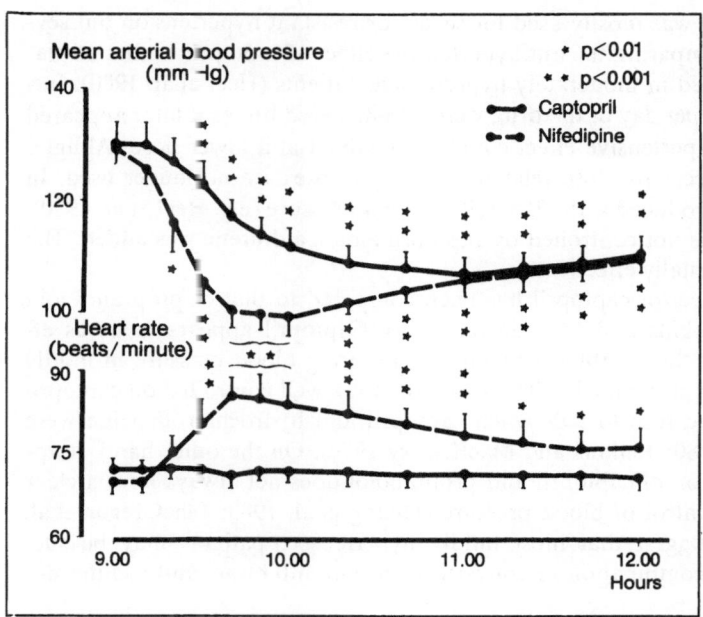

Fig. 1. Acute antihypertensive effect of a single dose of either captopril (1 mg/kg body weight) or nifedipine (20 mg) in hypertensive patients. From Soto et al. 1981.

effect of angiotensin II remains unchanged (Ferguson et al. 1977). The hypotensive effect of intravenous bradykinin is potentiated because ACE also inactivates bradykinin in blood and tissues (Erdos 1976).

Captopril (D3 mercapto-2-methylpropanoyl-1-proline) was the first orally active ACE inhibitor used in man and worldwide clinical experience of its use has already been obtained. MacGregor et al. (1981) showed that captopril lowers blood pressure in normotensive subjects. The hypotensive effect was primarily dependant on sodium balance. It was more pronounced in subjects on low sodium diet (19.6%) than in those having normal or high sodium intake where it averaged 16.5 and 11% respectively. In all groups of subjects, plasma aldosterone fell as a consequence of angiotensin II suppression. Urinary sodium excretion rose in subjects on normal or low sodium diets. These results show that a functional renin-angiotensin system is necessary to maintain blood pressure and sodium balance particularly when sodium intake is reduced.

In patients with mild hypertension, a single oral dose (1 mg/kg body weight) of captopril produced a fall in blood pressure which lasted more than 3 hours (Fig. 1) (Soto et al. 1981). In these patients, who had a normal sodium intake, maximal effect was observed after 90 minutes and averaged 17%. There was no change in heart rate. This constancy of heart rate despite a large fall in blood pressure has been observed in several studies (Fagard et al. 1979; Levenson et al. 1980) but is not well explained. It may be due to decreased baroreflex sensitivity, lack of increase in sympathetic nervous activity, increased vagal tone or decreased venous return. Heart rate and cardiac output also remain unchanged during short-term captopril treatment (Fagard et al. 1977).

119

As a new drug, captopril was mostly used for severe or resistant hypertension but several therapeutic trials comparing the antihypertensive effect of captopril to that of placebo have been performed in moderately hypertensive patients (Heel et al. 1980). Initially, more than 300 mg per day of the drug were administered but as it later appeared that a satisfactory antihypertensive effect could be obtained at a lower dose (Aldigier 1981) and since side-effects are dose related, such high doses are no longer used. In most studies, captopril produced a 15–25% fall in blood pressure (e.g. Heel et al. 1980). When blood pressure was not controlled by captopril alone, a diuretic was added. The combined therapy was usually effective.

The antihypertensive effect of captopril has been compared to that of propranol and hydrochlorothiazide (Jenkins and MacKinstry 1979). Captopril appears to be as efficient as the diuretic or the betablocker alone for lowering blood pressure in mildly hypertensive patients. Approximately 40% of patients were well controlled on captopril alone but this percentage rose to 90% when captopril and hydrochlorothiazide were combined (Heel et al. 1980; Jenkins and MacKinstry 1979). On the other hand, it appears that the combination of captopril and propranolol does not always have a clear additive effect on the control of blood pressure (Huang et al. 1980; MacGregor et al. 1982 a). These results suggest that most mildly hypertensive patients may be successfully treated with a combination of converting enzyme inhibitors and sodium depletion.

There was no correlation between the initial level of blood pressure and the response to converting enzyme inhibition in a group of moderately hypertensive patients (MacGregor et al. 1982 b).

The initial response of blood pressure to captopril appears to be related to plasma renin activity (Aldigier et al. 1981; Case et al. 1980; Soto et al. 1981; Weinberger 1980). However, such a correlation has not been found by all investigators, particularly when captopril is prescribed for long periods. It is likely that the magnitude of the initial fall in blood pressure observed in normotensive and hypertensive patients is primarily dependant on the suppression of angiotensin II. In high renin patients, such as those with renovascular hypertension or those treated with diuretics, the fall in blood pressure is more important than in low renin patients or in patients with primary aldosteronism. However, even in low renin essential hypertensive patients, converting enzyme inhibitors do lower blood pressure. It has been speculated that this effect may be due to factors other than angiotensin II suppression.

Several converting enzyme inhibitors other than captopril have been synthesized and some will probably become available for the treatment of hypertension. Enalapril (N[(S)-ethoxycarbonyl-3-phenylpropyl]-L-Alanyl-L-proline) is an orally active ACE inhibitor which is active over 24 hours and may be administered once a day (Patchett et al. 1980). When increasing amounts of Enalapril, within the range 1.25–20 mg, were given to patients with mild essential hypertension, a dose dependant decrease in blood pressure was observed. There was also a dose related effect on plasma aldosterone, plasma renin activity and potassium balance. The minimum dose of Enalapril able to maintain a blood pressure reduction of 10 mm Hg or more for 24 hours was found to be approximately 10 mg (Aldigier, personal communication).

As a consequence of the angiotensin II suppression, induced by acute administration of an ACE inhibitor, plasma renin activity rises and plasma aldosterone falls (Aldigier et al. 1981; Atlas et al. 1979). During short-term treatment there is also a decrease in angiotensinogen as a consequence of its consumption by renin and a slight increase in plasma potassium levels which can be correlated to the decrease in aldosterone (Aldigier et al. 1981; Clauser et al. 1982). During long-term treatment, plasma renin activity remains elevated but contradictory results have been obtained on plasma and urinary aldosterone and little information is available on potassium balance.

Renal blood flow and glomerular filtration rate are not decreased during converting enzyme blockade in man. In some studies, a slight increase in renal blood flow was observed (Mimran et al. 1979). Postural hypotension is usually not observed during ACE inhibitor therapy. However, in patients severely depleted by a diuretic or in those with accelerated hypertension and sodium loss, the fall in blood pressure is sometimes dramatic and postural hypotension may occur. Interruption of the renin-angiotensin system may cause renal insufficiency in patients who are sodium restricted and have bilateral renal artery stenosis or nephroangiosclerosis (Aldigier et al. 1982).

In summary, converting enzyme inhibitors lower blood pressure in hypertensive patients, without inducing tachycardia, postural hypotension, central side-effects or reduction in renal blood flow. In mild or moderate hypertension they seem to be effective either alone or in combination with diuretics. Inhibition of the renin-angiotensin system together with sodium depletion may control blood pressure in most patients with mild or moderate hypertension.

Calcium antagonists

Calcium antagonists interact with the so called 'slow channels' in the cell membrane and inhibit calcium influx into the cells. Several compounds with these properties have been synthesized and used as antiarrhythmic agents or coronary vasodilators but only three of them: verapamil, nifedipine and diltiaziem have been extensively studied in hypertension. Calcium antagonists are able to decrease vascular resistance and lower blood pressure in hypertensive patients. After acute administration of nifedipine (20 mg) to mildly hypertensive patients there was a rapid decrease in blood pressure, averaging 23%, after approximately 35 minutes (Fig. 1) (Soto et al. 1981). In this crossover study which was designed to compare the acute antihypertensive effect of a single dose of either nifedipine or captopril, nifedipine acted faster and gave a more pronounced decrease in the blood pressure. After 3 hours, however, blood pressure levels were identical with each treatment. As a consequence of sympathetic stimulation during the fall in blood pressure, heart rate rose after administration of nifedipine (Fig. 1). Calcium antagonists seem to be powerful antihypertensive agents in vasoconstricted patients. In hypertensive crises oral or sublingual nifedipine rapidly lowered blood pressure and decreased vascular resistance (Bertel et al. 1983). However, in normotensive subjects no significant changes in blood pressure were observed after verapamil, nifedipine or diltiaziem (Muiesan et al. 1981; Lederballe et al. 1980; Soto et al. 1981). MacGregor et al. (1982 b) showed that in patients with essential hypertension, the decrease in blood pressure after nifedipine was positively correlated with the initial level of blood pressure whereas the decrease in blood pressure after captopril was not. The results of these four studies suggest that the antihypertensive effect of calcium antagonists is primarily related to the absolute degree of arterial vasoconstriction. Several trials have been conducted with either verapamil or nifedipine in mildly or moderately hypertensive patients. In both short-term and long-term studies, the drugs were usually found to be efficient in lowering blood pressure (Spivak et al. 1983).

Bulher et al. (1982) gave verapamil to 43 patients with essential hypertension, age range 20–86, and treated them for up to 8 months. In 25 of these patients, verapamil at the appropriate dose was able to reduce diastolic blood pressure to less than 95 mm Hg. Some of these patients had been previously treated with either a betablocker or a diuretic. The antihypertensive effects of all 3 drugs in monotherapy were compared. Interestingly, the authors found that the decrease in blood pressure after verapamil was strongly correlated with the age of the patients. There was a negative correlation between pretreatment plasma renin activity and the fall in blood pressure but this may be explained by the well known relationship between age and plasma renin activity. Age was the strongest predictive factor for the antihypertensive effect of verapamil. A similar positive correlation between age and fall in blood pressure was observed for diuretics but a negative correlation was found for betablockers. On the basis of these data Bühler et al. (1982) proposed that calcium antagonists become an alternative choice to diuretics for the treatment of aged hypertensive patients.

Although both nifedipine and verapamil are calcium antagonists there may be differences between the haemodynamic effects of these drugs (Spivak et al. 1983). A short-term (2 weeks) trial compared the antihypertensive effect of verapamil (80–160 mg twice daily) to that of nifedipine (10–20 mg three times a day). The two drugs had identical effects on blood pressure (Lewis et al. 1981; Spivack et al. 1983). Heart rate was higher with nifedipine than with verapamil. This may be explained by the sympathetic stimulation induced by the fall in blood pressure. It has therefore been proposed that a betablocker, or clonidine or alpha-methyldopa might be added to nifedipine in order, at least partially, to oppose the effects of sympathetic stimulation. Moreover, propranolol has been shown to reduce side-effects in nifedipine-treated patients (Aoki et al. 1978). Verapamil has a more complex negative inotropic and chronotropic effect and tachycardia was not usually observed (Spivack et al. 1983).

Neither acute nor chronic administration of nifedipine appear to affect plasma renin activity (Oliver et al. 1979; Soto et al. 1981). An increase in plasma and urinary vasopressin was observed after acute administration of nifedipine probably as a result of the decrease in blood pressure and baroreflex stimulation (Soto et al. 1981).

In summary, calcium antagonists lower blood pressure in hypertensive patients. Although they have a powerful effect in severely vasoconstricted patients, making them useful drugs in the treatment of hypertensive emergencies, there is also evidence that calcium antagonists may control blood pressure in mild hypertension. They may be less active in young and moderately hypertensive than in old or severely hypertensive patients. More studies are needed to assess fully the antohypertensive effect of calcium antagonists in mild hypertension.

To complete this presentation on the new pharmacological approaches to the treatment of hypertension it should be mentioned that several groups have now synthesized direct renin inhibitors such as angiotensinogen analogues or pepstatin derivatives (Cody et al. 1980; Gardes et al. 1980). These compounds directly inhibit renin both *in vitro* and *in vivo* and reduce blood pressure in experimental high renin hypertension. Although they have so far only been used in animal models they might become new drugs for the specific inhibition of the renin-angiotensin system in man.

References

1 Aldigier JC, Plouin PF, Alexandre JM, Corvol P, Menard J (1981) Dose dependency of captopril effects in severely hypertensive patients. J Cardiovasc Pharmacol 3:1229-1235.
2 Aldigier JC, Plouin PF, Guyene TT, Thibonnier M, Corvol P, Menard J (1982) Comparison of the hormonal and renal effects of captopril in severe essential and renovascular hypertension. Am J Cardiol 49:1447-1452.
3 Alhenc-Gelas F, Plouin P-F, Ducrocq M-B, Corvol P, Menard J (1978) Comparison of the antihypertensive and hormonal effects of a cardioselective beta-blocker, acebutolol, and diuretics in essential hypertension. Am J Med 64:1005-1012.
4 Aoki K, Kondo Mochizaki A, Yoshida T, Kato S, Kato K, Takiwawa K (1978) Antihypertensive effect of Ca^{2+} antagonist in hypertensive patients in the absence and presence of beta adrenergic blockage. Am Heart J 96:218-226.
5 Atlas SA, Case DB, Sealey JE, Laragh JH, McKinstry DN (1979) Interruption of the renin-angiotensin system in hypertensive patients by captopril induces sustained reduction in aldosterone secretion, potassium retention and natriuresis. Hypertension 1:274-280.
6 Australian Therapeutic Trial in mild hypertension. Report by the Management Committee (1980) Lancet i: 1261-1267.
7 Bertel O, Conen D, Radu EW, Muller J, Lang C, Dubach UC (1983) Nifedipine in hypertensive emergencies. Br Med J 286:19-21.
8 Bühler FR, Hulthén UL, Kiowski W, Müller FB, Bolli P (1982) The place of the calcium antagonist verapamil in antihypertensive therapy. J Cardiovasc Pharmacol 4:S350-S357.
9 Case DB, Atlas SA, Laragh JH, Sullivan PA, Sealey JE (1980) Use of first-dose response or plasma renin activity to predict the long term effect of captopril: identification of triphasic pattern of blood pressure response. J Cardiovasc Pharmacol 2:339-346.
10 Clauser E, Genain C, Bouhnik, Corvol P, Menard J (1982) Variations de l'angiotensinogene et du des-angiotensine I-angiotensinogene chez l'homme et le rat au cours de l'inhibition de l'enzyme de conversion. Arch Mal Coeur n° Special; 157-161.
11 Cody RJ, Burton J, Evin G, Poulsen K, Herd JA, Haber E (1980) A substrate analog inhibitor of renin that is effective in vivo. Biochem Biophys Res Commun 97:230-235.
12 Cushman DW, Cheung HS, Sabo EF, Ondetti MA (1977) Design of potent competitive inhibitors of angiotensin-converting enzyme. Biochemistry 16:5484-5491.
13 Erdos EG (1976) Conversion of angiotensin I to angiotensin II. Am J Med 60:749-759.
14 Fagard R, Amery A, Lijnen P, Reybrouck T (1979) Haemodynamic effects of captopril in hypertensive patients comparison with saralasin. Clin Sci 57:131S-134S.
15 Ferguson RK, Brunner HR, Turini GA, Gavras H, McKinstry DN (1977) A specific orally active inhibitor of angiotensin converting enzyme in man. Lancet i:775-778.
16 Gardes J, Evin G, Castro B, Corvol P, Menard J (1980) Synthesis and renin inhibitory properties of a new soluble pepstatin derivative. J Cardiovasc Pharmacol 2:687-698.
17 Heel RC, Brodgen RN, Speight TM, Avery GS (1980) Captopril: a preliminary review of its pharmacological properties and therapeutic efficacy. Drugs 20:409-452.
18 Huang CM, Saloman J, Molteni A, Quintanilla A, De Greco F (1980) Antihypertensive effect of captopril and propranolol. Clin Pharmacol Ther 27:258-259.
19 Ibsen H, Rasmussen K, Jensen HAE, Leth A (1978) Changes in plasma volume and extracellular fluid volume after addition of hydralazine to propranolol in patients with hypertension. Acta Med Scand 203:419-423.
20 Jenkins AC, MacKinstry DN (1979) Review of clinical studies of hypertensive patients treated with captopril. Med J Aust 2: (Suppl 2) xxxii-xxxvii.
21 Laragh JH (1973) Vasoconstriction volume analysis for understanding and treating hypertension. The use of renin and aldosterone profiles. Am J Med 55:261-274.
22 Lederballe Petersen O, Christensen NJ, Rämsch KD (1980) Comparison of acute effects of nifedipine in normotensive and hypertensive man. J Cardiovasc Pharmacol 2:357-366.
23 Levenson J, Simon A, Tremmar M, Safar M (1980) Action antihypertensive du captopril: etude hemdynamique. Nouv Presse Med 9:617-619.
24 Lewis GRJ, Stewart DJ, Lewis BM, Bones PJ, Morley KD, Janus ED (1981) The antihypertensive effect of oral verapamil. Acute and long term administration and its effects on the high density lyoprotein values in plasma. In: Zanchetti and Kreber (eds) Calcium antagonism

in cardiovascular therapy. Experience with verapamil. Excerpta Medica, Amsterdam-Oxford-Princetown 270–277.

25 MacGregor GA, Markander ND, Roulston JA, Jones JC, Morton JJ (1981) The renin angiotensin system: a normal mechanism for maintaining blood pressure in normotensive and hypertensive subjects. In: Angiotensin converting enzyme inhibitors Morowitz ZP (ed) Urban and Swarzenberg-Baltimore 329–349.

26 MacGregor GA, Markandu ND, Banks RA, Bayliss J, Rouston JE, Jones JC (1982a) Captopril in essential hypertension contrasting effects of adding hydrochlorothiazide or propranolol. Br Med J 284:693–698.

27 MacGregor GA, Rotellar C, Markandu ND, Smith SS, Sagnella GA (1982b) Contrasting effects of nifedipine, captopril and propranolol in normotensive and hypertensive subjects. J Cardiovasc Pharmacol 4 (Suppl 3):S358–S362.

28 Maeda K, Takasugi T, Tsukano Y, Tanaka Y, Shiota K (1981) Clinical study on the hypertensive effect of diltiaziem hydrochloride. Int J Clin Pharmacol Therap Toxic 19:47–55.

29 Mimran A, Brunner HR, Turini GA, Waeber B, Brunner D (1979) Effect of captopril on renal vascular tone in patients with essential hypertension. Clin Sci 57:421S–432S

30 Muiesan G, Abigiti-Rosei E, Alicandri C, Bescki M, Castercano M, Corea L, Fariello R, Romanelli G, Pasini C, Platto L (1981) Influence of verapamil on catecholamines renin and aldosterone in essential hypertensive patients. In: Zanchetti and Krikler (eds) Calcium antagonism in cardiovascular therapy. Experience with verapamil. Excerpta Medica, Amsterdam-Oxford-Princeton 238–249.

31 Olivart MT, Bartorelli C, Polese A, Fiorentini O, Moruzzi P, Guazzi MD (1979) Treatment of hypertension with nifedipine, a calcium antagonistic agent. Circulation 59:1056–1062.

32 Soto ME, Thibonnier M, Sire O, Menard J, Corvol P, Milliez P (1981) Antihypertensive and hormonal effects of single oral doses of captopril and nifedipine in essential hypertension. Eur J Clin Pharmacol 20:157–161.

33 Spivack C, Ocken S, Frishman WH (1983) Calcium antagonists: clinical use in the treatment of systemic hypertension. Drugs: 25:154–177.

34 Triggle DJ, Swamy VC (1983) Calcium antagonists: some chemical-pharmacologic aspects. Circ Res 52 (Suppl 1):17–28.

35 Patchett AA, Harris E, Tristram E, et al. (1981) A new class of angiotensin – converting enzyme inhibitors. Nature 288:280–283.

36 Smith WM (1977) US Public Health Service Hospitals Cooperative Study Group. Treatment of mild hypertension. Results of ten year intervention trial. Circ Res 40 (Suppl i):98–105.

37 Veterans Administration Cooperative Study Group on antihypertensive agents. Effects of treatment on morbidity in hypertension. Results in patients with diastolic blood pressure averaging 90 through 114 mm Hg. JAMA 213C:1143–1152.

38 Weinberger MH (1980) Angiotensin converting enzyme (ACE 1) inhibition in treatment of resistant hypertension. Clin Pharmacol Ther 27:293.

Correspondence:
F. Alhenc-Gelas
Hopital Broussais
96, Rue Didot
75014 Paris
France

Discussion

McMAHON:
There are reports on the benefit of captopril in the treatment of mild hypertensives in whom renin levels are normal or low. You said that the degree of benefit correlated with the initial level of plasma renin activity. In theory I would agree but in practice it makes little difference what the renin level is.

ALHENC-GELAS:
If patients with low renin and those with high renin are included in the study group a correlation is observed. In a group of mildly hypertensive patients, there are many variables which mask such a correlation.

PEART:
There are problems in interpreting the actions of captopril and in being sure that they result from blocking angiotensin II as a pressor agent. I still think there is some doubt as to whether this is its only mode of action.

ALHENC-GELAS:
In some studies, the mildly hypertensive patients were on low sodium diets and hence had a higher plasma renin activity. In these cases there was a stronger correlation. I agree with you that low renin activity patients are still sensitive to converting enzyme inhibition which could indicate a completely different mechanism.

ESSE:
Can you envisage any advantage in using a renin inhibitor instead of a converting enzyme inhibitor in therapy?

ALHENC-GELAS:
I do not know if direct inhibitors of the renin-angiotensin system would be therapeutically useful.

PEART:
That question must be answered because better inhibitors are going to become available. I am impressed by how low plasma renin activity can be in people on certain doses of beta-blocker although blood pressure need not be lowered in these cirumstances. It seems to me that we have neglected to study a renin inhibitor which is already available.

ALHENC-GELAS:
There is some evidence that converting enzyme inhibitors may not completely block formation of angiotensin II. Maybe a more powerful inhibitor of angiotensin II formation is needed.

KOBINGER:
In pharmacological experiments the calcium antagonists have a marked negative inotropic effect on the myocardium. Did you notice signs of cardiac insufficiency in elderly patients?

ALHENC-GELAS:
No.

McMAHON:
Do you prefer to use a drug like nifedipine with a beta-blocker rather than verapamil which inhibits the SA node and the AV node?

ALHENC-GELAS:

There are arguments in favour of both drugs. Nifedipine has less effect on atrioventricular conduction but increases sympathetic activity so one would probably have to prescribe a beta-blocker at the same time. Verapamil does not have this effect. In a study with a one year follow-up period there have been no dramatic side-effects or complications with verapamil.

PEART:

Verapamil has an even greater effect upon the heart than does nifedipine despite the fact that most studies of nifedipine show an increased cardiac output. I take that to mean that the peripheral resistance is markedly reduced by nifedipine. Despite that, nifedipine is an excellent drug for the prevention of angina.

KOBINGER:

That might be the case where the heart is completely normal. What about elderly patients with borderline cardiac insufficiency? In our laboratory we have noted a correlation between the negative inotropic effect and the vascular relaxing effect of calcium antagonists.

General discussion

FRANKLIN:
In the hypertension and follow-up program where maximum effort was made to ensure compliance in the step-care group there was still a sizeable group of patients who did not take the drugs. There is certainly a hard core group of patients who defy our ability to persuade them of the importance of antihypertensive therapy.

PEART:
There are other studies which show that drugs given three times a day are less likely to be taken that those given once a day.

HAYDUK:
The hypertension detection and follow-up study shows a low treatment effect in men below the age of 50. An as yet unpublished German study shows that this group have the poorest compliance. There could be a correlation between these two results.

DRAYER:
I am not sure that there is conclusive evidence for the general statements we make about compliance and the doctor-patient relationship or the frequency of drug administration. Studies of compliance do not tend to find definitive explanations of who is and who is not compliant.

McMAHON:
Compliance has been improved in the last few years with the advent of once or twice daily medication. Clearly written instructions are also important. It is very easy to forget whether you took the morning or evening dose but easy to remember whether you have changed a transdermal system because of the pale patch it leaves on the skin.

WEBER:
In the Australian study of the frequency of side-effects in different treatment groups the people in active therapy have only slightly more side-effects than those who knew they were getting no treatment at all. All three groups had a significantly higher frequency of complaints than normotensive volunteers in a parallel study group. One is left with the impression that hypertensives as a group are more susceptible to complaints of depression, drowsiness and difficulties with sexual activity. It is perhaps not surprising that compliance is not good in a group who are having to confront the psychological problem induced by being told that they have a chronic condition. There is probably a certain amount of denial. I am sure that the issue of compliance is not only a problem of education or of simplicity of treatment. We are dealing with something fundamentally more difficult than that and I do not know whether there is a simple answer.

PEART:
The side-effect issue itself is a very important one to which we should address ourselves. There are some people who do not like taking pills of any sort. We are talking about subjects who have no symptoms to start with. If the treatment you introduce has effects which the subject does not like, he or she will stop taking it. You will not necessarily find out why unless you are very persistent in asking them questions about their life in general. It was in this way that we succeeded in discovering a number of side-effects of which we had not been aware. For example, the effect of thiazides in causing impotence. It was only when we followed this up properly with a placebo group that the difference emerged.

McMAHON:
One part of the problem of compliance is side-effects, the other part is efficacy. Patients need to be educated about their disease. Most American practitioners do not have time for the education required. The clinics which are most successful are those with paramedical people who can explain to patients the consequences of not taking their medication. I had a 22-year-old patient who became impotent on thiazides and who chose to remain on the treatment because his mother died of a stroke and his father had severe malignant hypertension. He chose to be impotent.

PEART:
You mean you haven't got him on clonidine?

McMAHON:
No, he was only on thiazides.

FRANKLIN:
Another useful technique to improve compliance is teaching patients to take their own blood pressure at home. This reinforces the importance of taking their drugs because they can see the improvement in their blood pressure levels.

Advances in treatment

Chairman: M. P. Sambhi

Rate-controlled drug delivery and the reduction of risk

K. Heilmann

There are several drugs which would not be on the market today were it not for their associated delivery systems. An old, but very good, example is the inhalation anaesthetic halothane. To use it safely requires a special vaporizer which enables the anaesthetist to 'dial' a fixed concentration of the agent in the patient's inspired air. This delivery system not only makes halothane simpler to use than other agents, but also gives it a safety margin which it would not have if given by the open-drop inhalation method (which worked quite well for ether). Also, the halothane vaporizer has been used very artfully in promotion to persuade anaesthetists to use the new product. Today, 25 years after its introduction, halothane dominates the inhalation anaesthetic market in all technologically advanced countries, and the vaporizer has become an integral part of contemporary anaesthetic practice.

Transdermal nitroglycerin

Most of the major pharmaceutical companies are active in the delivery systems field. The advent of transdermal delivery of nitroglycerin is a good example of an old drug which has to some extent been rediscovered. Research carried out in the past decade with modern methods has led to new uses for the drug in cardiac care and a greater understanding of the drug's pharmacokinetic and pharmacodynamic behaviour. With this has come a recognition that there is a major market for a truly effective agent capable of preventing anginal attacks instead of merely relieving the symptoms. It is, however, too soon to know if this emphasis on prevention will favourably alter the natural history and progression of ischaemic heart disease. It is not unreasonable to infer that the ability of continuously administered nitroglycerin to prevent many episodes of oxygen deprivation may slow or arrest the progression to congestive heart failure. That proposition has to be tested, however, and would involve a clinical trial of formidable dimensions.

The potential of drug delivery systems

The pharmaceutical industry is still assimilating the effects of the thalidomide disaster of 1962. There has been a sharp drop in the flow of new products based on new chemical agents and a sharp escalation in both the timescale and costs of developing pharmaceutical products. Delivery systems are now generally seen to provide the following antidotes to this difficult situation.

131

Table 1. Advantages of drug delivery systems

Realization of defined temporal patterns of drug release and concentration
Reduction of quantity of drug required for efficacious therapy
Reduction of side-effects
Improvement of drug safety
Improved opportunity for patient compliance
Feasibility of routine therapy with substances having short biological half-lives

---

1. They provide a way of improving drug administration by means of less frequent dosing, fewer or less severe side-effects, and sometimes improved round-the-clock efficacy. Drug delivery systems certainly offer the opportunity to improve patient compliance by reducing some problems connected with conventional forms of drug administration. All compliance studies make clear that reducing the frequency of daily drug administration substantially improves compliance. Also, since non-compliance correlates closely with the type, severity and frequency of undesirable drug effects, it is fair to assume that patient compliance may be increased by reducing side-effects.
2. Delivery systems can sometimes make wholly new products out of existing drugs without the formidably long periods needed to develop new chemical agents. The transdermal delivery of nitroglycerin, for example, makes it possible for the first time to prolong the effect of a single dose of the drug over a period of 24 hours. It is a major step forward both in technology and therapy.
3. Delivery systems can do just what the special vaporizer did for halothane: they can add an important margin of safety; they can also guard against non-compliance, since transdermal delivery systems, for example, can last as long as a week, irrespective of whether the half-life of the agent being delivered is minutes or hours.
Drug delivery systems now offer us the possibility of delivering a drug continuously over a given period, in some cases to a single target organ. These possibilities, created by technology that now appears to be virtually unlimited in its application, offer a precision of drug administration that conventional forms of drug administration cannot match. Drug delivery systems offer maximum efficacy, selectivity and safety, and have a number of other important advantages, as shown in Table 1.

Pharmacodynamics

The ideas of a new science called pharmacodynamics are entering into the assessment of new drugs, both in animal and clinical testing programmes. If the details of a pharmacodynamic study of a drug are to be put to practical use, delivery systems must be available at all levels of drug research and development. That condition is now met, or is at least close to being met. A knowledge of pharmacodynamics makes it clear that certain quantitative aspects of a drug's actions should be understood before the dose form/delivery system is chosen for the final product. This principle contradicts conventional wisdom and practice in pharmaceutical research and development, which says that testing should be done first with a conventional dose form (i.e. one which incorporates no kinetic specifications on the rate at which the drug is released *in vivo*). Developments in pharmacodynamics provide a better way to use the results of animal studies to design the first human trials. The strengthening of this weak link in the development of new chemical agents is one of the most important implications of delivery systems in the medium-to-long term.

The future of drug delivery systems

Drug safety requires the producer to comply with legal regulations aimed at minimizing the risks of drug use in man. Drug delivery systems have shown that drug risk can also be minimized by a new technological route: by controlling drug delivery via a special drug delivery system.

Any pharmaceutical product is truly successful when physicians recognize it as effective and safe and patients accept it and use it properly. Reduction of the symptoms of disease, accompanied by minimal complaints and side-effects, in other words minimal burden on the patient, provides a direct measure of the worth of a product. Reaching this goal is often difficult or impossible; many agents require frequent application and cause side-effects potent enough to interfere with the patient's work or quality of life. Drugs on the market with considerable therapeutic potential are frequently not used or under used because therapy would be too complex or burdensome for the patient. The overall effectiveness of an agent correlates directly with its dose form, a fact which has in recent years directed interest towards optimizing drug action through new forms of dosing. Perhaps by the end of this decade it will be the rule, rather than the exception, for new drugs to appear first in a 'delivery system', with the dose rate specified not by the total quantity of drug, but by the rate of delivery to the body.

References

1 Heilmann K (1982) Therapeutische Systeme. 3rd Edition. Enke F. Stuttgart.
2 Heilmann K (1983) Therapeutic Systems. 2nd Edition. Thieme-Stratton New York
3 Urquhart J (ed.) (1981) Controlled-release pharmaceuticals. American Pharmaceutical Association, Washington. (A French edition is available from Editions Sante, 19 Rue Louis-le-Grand, Paris 75002.)
4 James BG (1982) The Marketing of Generic Drugs: a guide to counterstrategies for the technology intensive pharmaceutical companies. Associated Business Press, London. Scrip Bookshop, Richmond, England.

Correspondence:
K. Heilmann, M. D.
Technical University, Munich
University of California, Los Angeles, USA
Beethovenplatz 2–3
8000 Munich 2
FRG

Clonidine rate – controlled system: technology and kinetics

J. E. Shaw, D. Enscore and L. Chu

Introduction

Clonidine is a potent, centrally acting hypotensive agent, available commercially in tablet form, for oral administration (Catapres®, Boehringer Ingelheim Ltd.). Oral doses of 0.2–1.5 mg administered b.d. or t.d.s., to give plasma clonidine concentrations in the range of 0.3–5.0 ng/ml, have been found satisfactory for the control of blood pressure.

A transdermal dosage form for this antihypertensive agent must provide the following three characteristics: a hypotensive action at least equal to that of the oral drug, side-effect reduction and a simplified medication regimen. Clonidine is an excellent candidate for transdermal therapy; it has sufficient potency and appropriate physico-chemical properties. Moreover, a strong medical rationale exists for its administration in a manner that will maximise compliance as the hypertensive patient's regimen must necessarily be lifelong. Fluctuations in plasma levels with oral drug administration have been associated with unwanted side-effects, particularly drowsiness and dry mouth (Black 1983; Mroczek et al. 1982). Rate-controlled, continuous administration of clonidine should provide the opportunity for equally effective blood pressure control with minimal side-effects.

Prior to the advent of the recent transdermal drug delivery systems, the most widely used method of delivering drugs topically for systemic therapy was to apply ointments to intact skin. With this mode drug administration large variations in the rate and extent of drug absorption can occur due to differences in the intrinsic permeability of skin, as well as differences brought about by the vehicle formulation. Indeed, the effects of skin site (Feldman and Maibach 1967; Shaw and Chandrasekaran 1981), condition (Mroczek 1983), age (Mroczek 1983; Feldman and Maibach 1965), sex (Shaw and Chandrasekaran 1981), metabolism (Mroczek 1983) and temperature (Shaw and Chandrasekaran 1981) on percutaneous drug absorption have been well documented. Keeping all else constant, the mass of ointment used and area of skin to which the ointment is applied can be varied unintentionally. These two factors affect the drug plasma concentration achieved, and the length of time for which effective plasma levels are maintained (Kirby and Woods 1981). Use of skin as a reproducible route of entry of drugs into the bloodstream requires an understanding of the barrier properties of the skin; in addition, it requires that control over the rate of drug delivery to the systemic circulation reside in the dosage form, and not in the skin.

ALZA Corporation, in collaboration with Boehringer Ingelheim, has developed a transdermal therapeutic system (clonidine TTS) for controlled delivery of clonidine to the systemic circulation. This is a small, flexible system of membranes that adheres comfortably to the skin. After placement of the system on the skin surface, the drug diffuses from the system through the skin, and is absorbed into the bloodstream and distributed throughout the body.

The performance of the transdermal dosage form has been evaluated both *in vitro* and *in vivo,* with emphasis placed on bioavailability of drug from the system, efficacy of the drug programme, and topical safety of the dosage form.

Dosage form design

Clonidine TTS is a film 0.2 mm thick, composed of four layers (Fig. 1): a backing layer that provides a physical barrier to loss of clonidine: a reservoir that provides for a continuous supply of drug for one week; a microporous control membrane that controls the rate of delivery of clonidine from the drug reservoir to the skin surface; and an adhesive formulation containing clonidine. The drug in the adhesive provides the initial input of clonidine necessary for saturation of the skin binding sites at the initiation of therapy; this adhesive layer also permits passage of the drug and provides effective attachment to the skin. Prior to use, a protective release liner, covering the adhesive layer, is removed and discarded.

The dosage form is designed to provide rate-controlled, continuous administration of drug over 7 days. Figure 2 illustrates the rate of release of clonidine from the transdermal system *in vitro,* using water, at 32 °C, as the receptor solution. It is evident that the rate of release of drug from the system is approximately 5 times greater in the first 0–8 hours, when the drug is being released from the adhesive, than the rate of release during the remainder of the 168 hour lifetime of the system, when the drug released comes from the reservoir.

In vivo studies

Two studies in normal male volunteers have provided evidence for the bioavailability of clonidine administered transdermally from clonidine TTS.

First study

In the first study, each subject received oral clonidine (0.1 mg b.d.) for 4 days, and two clonidine TTS (2×2.5 cm^2 to give a total area of application of 5 cm^2) for 7 days. Order of treatments was randomized.

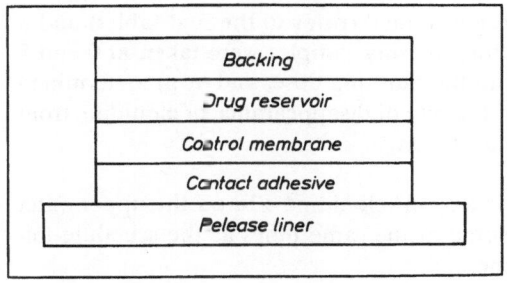

| Backing |
| Drug reservoir |
| Control membrane |
| Contact adhesive |
| Release liner |

Fig. 1. Cross-sectional diagram of clonidine TTS (drawing not to scale)

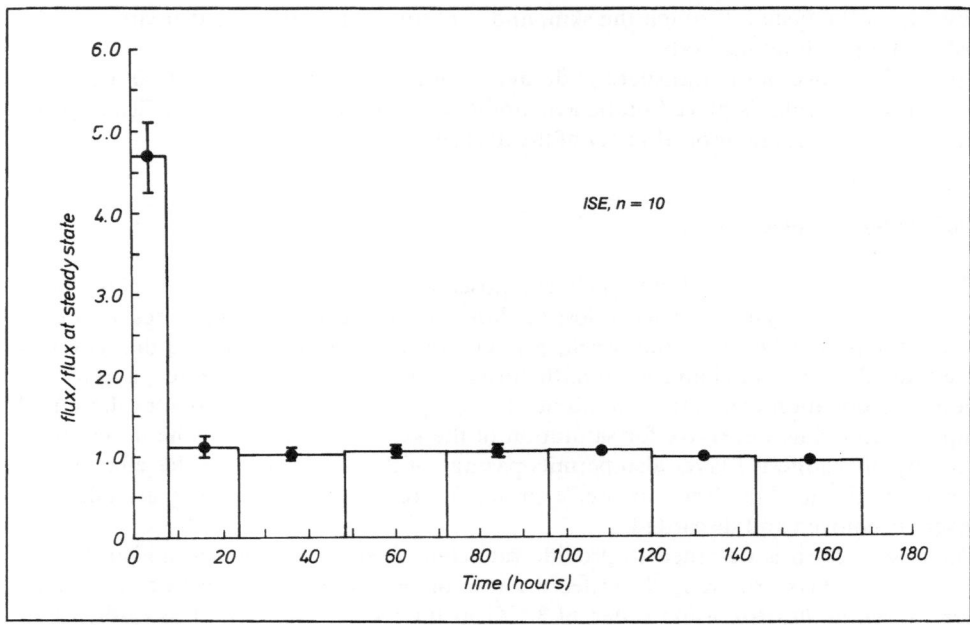

Fig. 2. *In vitro* drug release rate from clonidine TTS

Seventeen healthy male volunteers aged 21–38 years participated in this two-part, open label, cross-over study. All subjects gave their informed consent to participate. A complete medical history was obtained and a physical examination was performed including electrocardiogram, blood chemistry profile and urinalysis on each candidate. Prior to entry in the study, subjects were evaluated for their ability to tolerate the pharmacological effects of clonidine by administering an oral dose of clonidine hydrochloride (0.1 mg); blood pressure, heart rate and other pharmacological effects were monitored before and after clonidine administration. Subjects were requested to abstain from alcohol and other drugs beginning 24 hours before the study and continuing throughout the study period.

a) Oral clonidine: Each subject was given 0.1 mg clonidine hydrochloride every 12 hours for 4 days. Plasma samples were taken at time 0 (prior to the first tablet) and 8 hours thereafter. On days 2 and 3 of the study, plasma samples were taken at 0 and 8 hours, and on day 4, every 2 hours following the morning dose, and at predetermined times throughout days 5 and 6 to determine the rate of disappearance of clonidine from the plasma following administration of the last tablet.

b) Transdermal clonidine: Each subject wore a 5 cm² clonidine TTS on the upper outer arm. Plasma levels of clonidine were measured at the same times as the schedule followed during administration of oral clonidine.

Blood pressure and heart rate were measured daily throughout the periods of drug administration, in the sitting and standing positions after the subject had rested for at least five minutes. Blood pressures were taken in triplicate in each position and the mean of the three readings was recorded. Subjects were questioned regarding the appearance of any other pharmacological effects. All subjects who entered completed both phases of this study.

With oral clonidine, 0.1 mg every 12 hours, plasma levels attained a steady C_{min} value of approximately 400 pg/ml (Figure 3) by third day of drug administration. On the 4th day of the study, the mean peak plasma level achieved, 2 hours after drug administration, was 789 pg/ml (Figure 4), giving a mean C_{max} to C_{min} ratio of approximately two. The rate of disappearance of clonidine from the plasma following the last oral dose (mean half life, 11 hours) was consistent with the reported properties of the drug.

With transdermal administration of clonidine, the plasma levels gradually increased following placement of the system on the upper outer arm, and attained a steady state value in 2–3 days of approximately 400 pg/ml (Figure 3). The constancy of drug input was reflected in the constancy of the plasma levels maintained on the fourth day of wearing the clonidine TTS (Figure 4). The C_{max} to C_{min} value was one. Plasma levels were maintained for 8 hours following removal of the clonidine TTS, and then declined slowly during the subsequent 2 days.

Analysis of the area under the plasma curve (AUC) on day 4 of drug administration indicated that wearing of clonidine TTS, 5 cm² in area, provided an AUC that was equivalent to 76% of the AUC attained with oral administration of 0.2 mg clonidine hydrochloride per day. A decrease in both systolic and diastolic blood pressures was noted in these normal healthy volunteers with administration of clonidine via both the

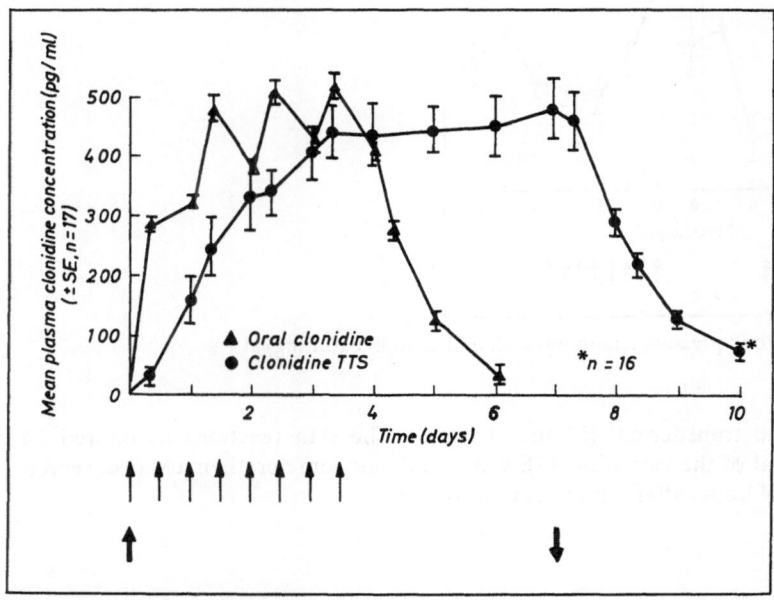

Fig. 3. Plasma clonidine levels during clonidine administration. Clonidine TTS (5 cm²) applied ↑, removed ↓. Oral clonidine (0.1 mg) at ↑

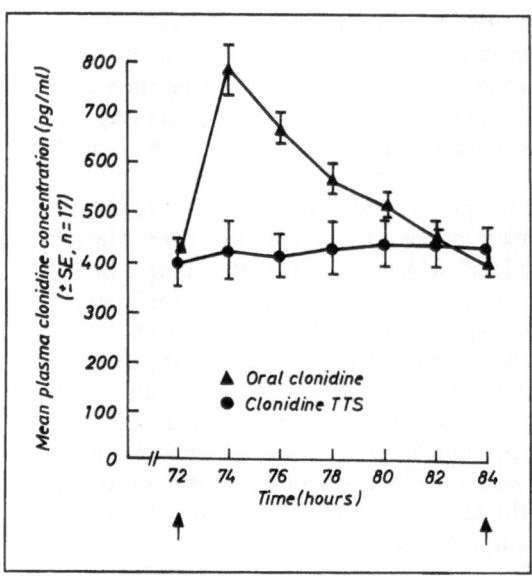

Fig. 4. Plasma clonidine levels on day 4 of study. Clonidine TTS (5 cm²) and oral clonidine (0.1 mg) at ↑

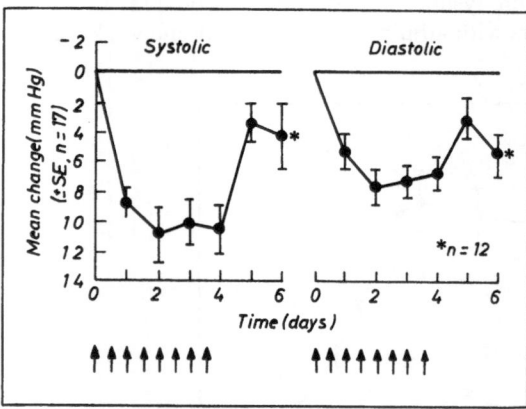

Fig. 5. Changes in blood pressure (standing) with oral clonidine (0.1 mg) at ↑

oral (Figure 5) and transdermal (Figure 6) routes. The skin reactions monitored 24 hours after removal of the clonidine TTS were minimal; some erythema was observed but faded within 24 hours after removal of the system.

Second study

In the second study we evaluated the relationship of clonidine plasma levels at steady state (120, 144, and 168 hours after system application) to four different sizes of cloni-

138

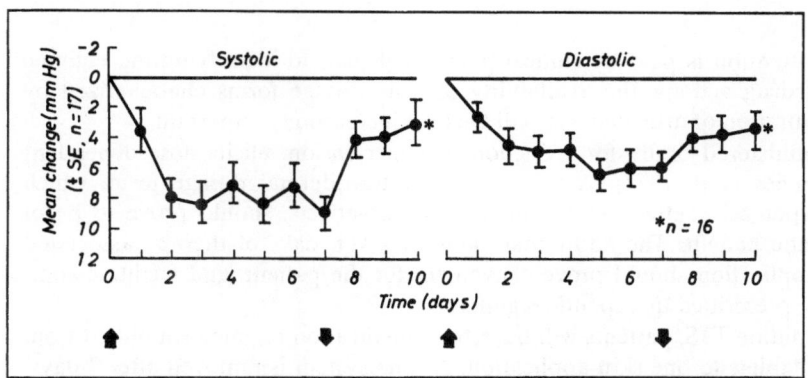

Fig. 6. Changes in blood pressure (standing) with clonidine TTS (5 cm²) applied ⬆, removed ⬇

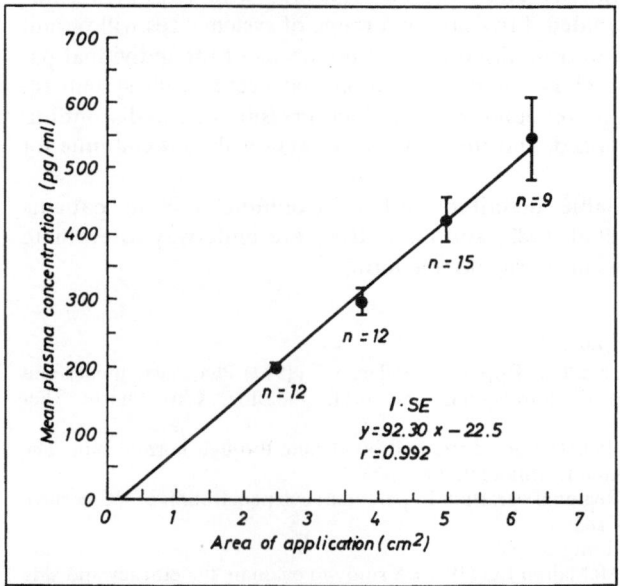

Fig. 7. Effect of area of application of clonidine TTS on steady state plasma clonidine concentration (120, 144, 168 hours)

dine TTS (2.5, 3.75, 5.0, and 6.25 cm² in area). All systems were placed on the upper outer arm of normal volunteers for 7 days, and plasma levels of clonidine were measured throughout the 7 day wearing. Following removal, the transdermal systems were analyzed for residual drug content. Knowing the mean initial drug content of the systems, the amount of drug available to the systemic circulation was calculated. This was shown to be a direct function of the area of the system worn (Figure 7). Following removal of the systems, plasma levels again remained constant for at least 8 hours. Thereafter, plasma levels began to decrease; at 32 hours following system removal they were approximately one-half of the steady-state values.

Conclusions

As increasing attention is paid by clinical pharmacologists to identifying the regimen dependence of drug actions, the availability of drug dosage forms characterized by their rate and duration of drug delivery will become increasingly important.

Clonidine, administered orally for reduction of hypertension, elicits dose dependent side-effects (Davies et al. 1977). A rate-controlled transdermal dosage form, which maintains a hypotensive effect while minimizing side-effects, should prove to be of major therapeutic benefit. The additional value of seven days of therapy associated with a single application should prove convenient for the patient, and facilitate compliance with the prescribed therapeutic regimen.

With use of clonidine TTS, patients will have their medication regimen simplified from 14 weekly oral tablets to one skin application. As one system is removed after 7 days' wearing it is recommended that a second system be immediately placed on a fresh skin site. The therapeutic concentrations of drug in plasma will be continuously maintained, and the sharp peaking concentrations, known to be associated with unwanted pharmacological effects, should be avoided. Provision of a range of system sizes will permit convenient and flexible titration of drug input rates to the needs of the individual patient. The gradual fall in plasma clonidine concentration that occurs after system removal has two advantages: abrupt 'rebound' rises in blood pressure due to discontinuation of treatment may be minimized, and the hypotensive action should continue for some time.

Preliminary data is now available describing use of clonidine TTS in patients (Michaels et al. 1983; Mroczek et al. 1982) and many trials are underway to evaluate both the efficacy and safety of this new drug dosage form.

References

1 Black CD (1983) U S Pharm 7 (11):49.
2 Davies DS, Wing LMH, Reid JL, Neill E, Tippett P, Dollery CT (1977) Pharmacokinetics and concentration-effect relationships of intravenous and oral clonidine. Clin Pharm Ther 21:593–601.
3 Feldman RJ, Maibach HI (1965) Penetration of ^{14}C hydrocortisone through normal skin. The effect of stripping and occlusion. Arch Dermatol 91:661–666.
4 Feldman RJ, Maibach HI (1967) Regional variation in percutaneous penetration of ^{14}C cortisol in man. J Invest Dermatol 48:181–183.
5 Kirby JA, Woods SL (1981) Heart Lung 10 (5).
6 Michaels RC, Jain AK, Ryan JR, McMahon FG (1983) A study to evaluate the efficacy and side effects of clonidine TTS as initial therapy in mild hypertension. Clin Pharm Ther 33:229.
7 Mroczek WJ (1982) Skin route cuts clonidine side effects. Med World News 23 (11):85.
8 Mroczek WJ, Ulrych MD, Yoder RN (1982) Weekly transdermal clonidine administration in hypertensive patients. Clin Pharm Ther 31:252.
9 Shaw JE, Chandrasekaran SK (1981) Transdermal therapeutic systems. In: Prescott LF and Nimmo WS (Eds) Drug absorption. The proceedings of the International Conference on Drug Absorption, Edinburgh, September 1979. ADIS Press, Balgowlah, Australia 186–193.

Correspondence:
Dr. J. E. Shaw
ALZA Corporation
950 Page Mill Road
P.O. Box 10950
Palo Alto
California 94303-0802
U.S.A.

Discussion

FRANKLIN:
You have shown that a constant clonidine level of 400 pg/ml achieved a good blood pressure reduction but have you explored a lower level, for example 300 pg/ml?

SHAW:
We have not done that. The aim of the study that I have described was to achieve an understanding of how the system works and to relate that to the administration of the drug. It was not really designed to look at blood pressure and it was not a placebo-controlled study. We simply monitored the blood pressure to look at the safety of the subject. There have been, and still are, extensive clinical trials looking at the rate of drug input which effectively lowers blood pressure in the hypertensive patient. We will hear about this later from Dr Weber. In these clinical studies the level that is appropriate for the individual patient has been found by titration.

DRAYER:
Were your studies on skin absorption done with cadaver skin and do you have any evidence that the results hold for living man?

SHAW:
Yes. The reason for that is that the stratum corneum is the barrier and even in the living the stratum corneum is a layer of dead keratinized epithelial cells.

DRAYER:
I have heard a dermatologist say that a high concentration of drug might be built up beneath the skin and is released more slowly than one might expect on the basis of blood flow through that area. This could delay release of the drug.

SHAW:
The control lies in the dosage formula. A gradient of drug concentration through the skin is established with the highest concentration being in the upper layers of the stratum corneum. The skin has a rich blood flow which can carry away all the drugs delivered in the vicinity of the vessels.

MATHIAS:
You have shown that the relationship between clonidine level and blood pressure was fairly stable over the study period. What about side-effects? Were they reduced in the transdermal phase compared with the oral studies?

SHAW:
A number of our volunteers were very sleepy in the afternoon on oral clonidine but were functioning quite well with the patch. However it is difficult to draw firm conclusions as our study was not placebo-controlled.

SAMBHI:
Is it advisable to look for a non-hairy part of the skin or does it not matter?

SHAW:
It does not matter with respect to absorption of the drug and a steady-state input into the systemic circulation, as there is little movement through the sweat glands or the hair follicles, but it is important to ensure good contact between the adhesive surface of the system and the skin.

SAMBHI:
Would you shave hairy patients?

SHAW:
No. Shaving will inevitably strip off the stratum corneum which will interfere with the performance of the system, because the capacity of the skin for maintaining drug gradients will be altered.

HAYDUK:
Dr Heilmann, could you tell me how much clonidine is given into the eye and how much is absorbed?

HEILMANN:
It is thought that drug treatment on the eye is local drug treatment but this is not true. About two-thirds of the drug administered to the eye is absorbed. Plasma clonidine levels may be in the same range as that found during oral dosage for blood pressure treatment. Doses which can effectively lower blood pressure also effectively lower intraocular pressure by vasoconstriction in the eye.

PEART:
Which vessels does clonidine act upon to cause vasoconstriction in the eye? Are we talking about scleral veins?

HEILMANN:
No, the choroidal vessels.

Absorption of clonidine from a transdermal therapeutic system when applied to different body sites

K. Hopkins[1], L. Aarons[2] and M. Rowland[2]

Catapres-TTS® is a transdermal therapeutic system for clonidine. The device is a circular unit, composed of a flexible system of membranes, which adheres to the skin. Clonidine, released from the system at a controlled rate, is absorbed through the skin and distributes throughout the body. The current device is a 7-day system aimed at providing a relatively stable plasma concentration of clonidine, with the objective of optimising efficacy and patient compliance whilst minimising associated side effects.

The success of the transdermal system depends on the release of drug from the system being the controlling step in the absorption of drug into the body. This criterion is more likely to be met if the skin is highly permeable to the drug. The permeability of the skin to substances varies widely between different regions of the body (Feldman et al. 1967). The current recommended site of application of Catapres-TTS is the upper outer arm. With the idea of minimising repeated covering of a particular area of skin, the present study was designed to investigate whether the release of clonidine is affected by the site of application of the transdermal system. The sites chosen for investigation were the upper outer arm (reference), the upper outer thigh, and the chest. Reported here are preliminary findings based on measurement of clonidine in plasma and in the used transdermal system.

Methods

The study received the approval of a local Ethical Committee. The trial was randomized and open-labelled. Three application sites were used: upper outer arm, upper outer thigh and chest. The system was 3.75 cm² in size and contained 2.64 mg of clonidine, designed to deliver approximately 9.56 µg clonidine/hour for 7 days. Non-hairy sites were selected in almost all subjects but the chest of one very hairy male had to be shaved 24 hours before the investigation commenced.

Twelve healthy volunteers (three females and nine males; age range 21–40 years; weight range 54–89 kg) with no skin disease and no history of skin allergy, took part in the study. Each volunteer gave their written informed consent.

The protocol involved a 7-day application followed by a 7-day washout period and lasted for 6 weeks. The transdermal system was applied at 09.00 hours on the first day of each treatment period. Blood samples were taken immediately before application, and at 14.00 and 18.00 hours on each subsequent day a blood sample was taken at

1 Medical Unit, Medeval Ltd., Coupland III, University of Manchester, Manchester, M13 9PL, England
2 Department of Pharmacy, University of Manchester, Manchester M13 9PL, England

18.00 hours, except at weekends. The total 24-hour urine production was also collected. After removal, the used system was returned to Boehringer Ingelheim (Germany) for analysis by hplc, of the residual clonidine. The concentration of clonidine in plasma was determined by radioimmunoassay (Arndts et al., 1981). Blood pressure and pulse rate were monitored for safety reasons.

Results and Discussion

The system remained in position extremely well throughout the trial; there was only one instance of a system becoming partly detached. Changes in blood pressure and pulse rate were minimal during application of the transdermal system.

Figures 1 and 2 illustrate differences between subjects on the influence of site of application of the transdermal system on the plasma clonidine concentration-time profile. In one subjects no differences are seen between sites of skin application (Fig. 1), whereas clear differences exist in another subject (Fig. 2), with highest concentrations being seen after application of the system to the chest and lowest when the upper outer thigh was used. The latter subject was the one in whom the chest site was shaved, which may explain the early rapid rise in plasma-clonidine seen when this site was used.

Figure 3 summarises the mean plasma clonidine concentration data for the three treatment sites for all 12 subjects. Clear differences are seen, with the plasma clonidine concentration being highest when the transdermal system is applied to the chest and lowest when applied to the upper outer thigh.

The elimination half-life of clonidine is approximately 24 hours (Arndts et al., 1983), and it is therefore anticipated, on pharmacokinetic grounds, that a plateau drug concentration will be reached in approximately 4 days (4 half-lives) following a constant rate of drug input. The present data confirm this expectation. The plasma concentration was slightly higher on day 6 than on day 3 after the application, for all three skin

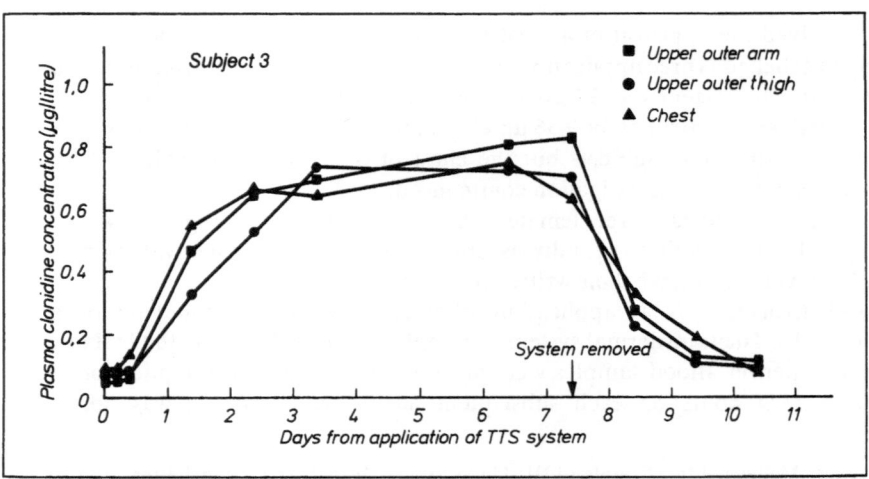

Fig. 1. No differences are seen in the plasma clonidine concentration for subject 3, when clonidine-transdermal system is applied to different skin sites.

144

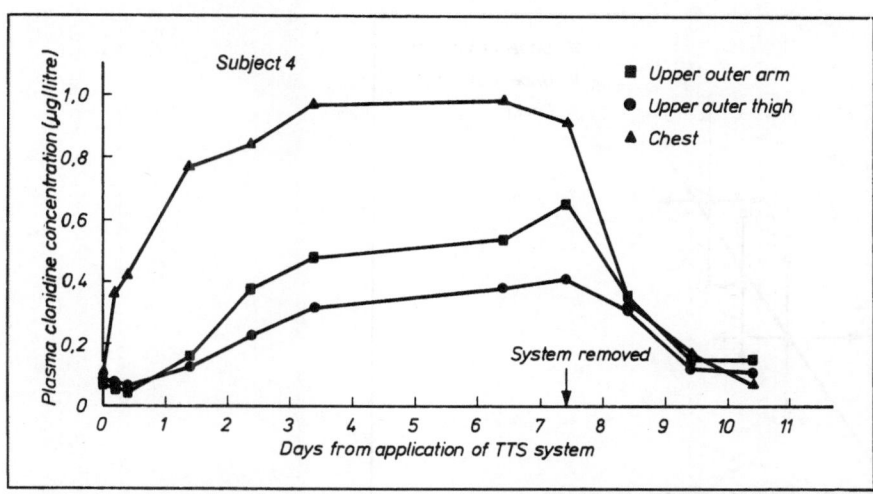

Fig. 2. In subject 4, the plasma clonidine concentration is highest following application of clonidine-transdermal system to the chest and lowest when applied to the upper outer thigh.

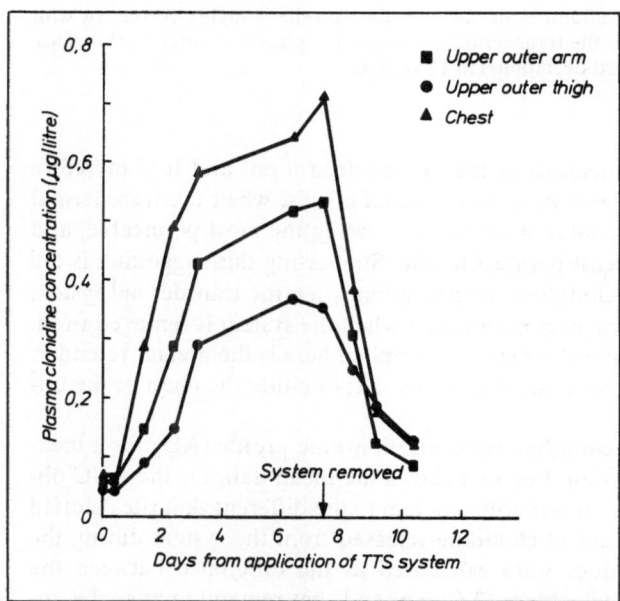

Fig. 3. Graph showing the mean plasma clonidine concentration against time during application of the transdermal system, and its removal from different skin sites.

sites, but no statistically significant differences were found between the plasma concentration on days 6 and 7. The mean of the results on days 6 and 7 were therefore taken as an estimate of the plateau concentration. Significant differences in the plateau concentration between all three sites of application were observed, the order being chest > upper outer arm > upper outer thigh.

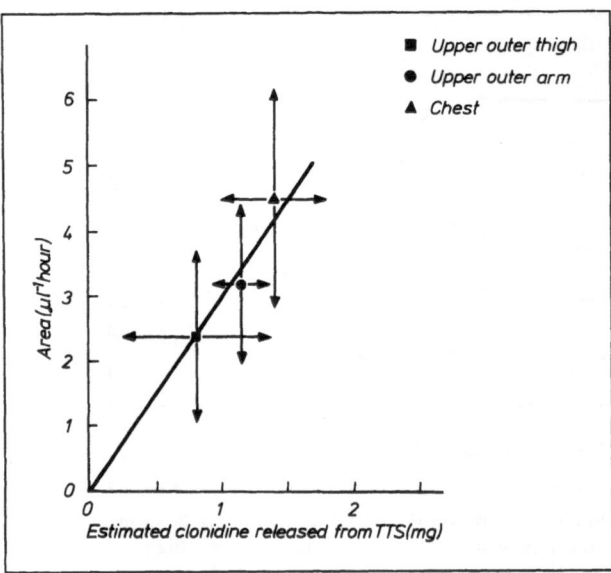

Fig. 4. The area under the plasma clonidine concentration-time profile is highly correlated with the amount of clonidine released from the transdermal system, when placed at different skin sites. Shown are the mean data (and standard deviations) in 12 volunteers.

The plateau concentration is a measure of the rate of drug input and it is therefore concluded that *differences in the rate of input of clonidine* exist when the transdermal system is applied to different skin sites, with the chest being the most permeable, and the upper outer thigh being the least permeable, site. Supporting this suggestion is the more *sluggish rise* in the plasma clonidine concentration when the transdermal system is applied to, and the *slower decline* in concentration when the system is removed from, the upper outer thigh as against the chest (Fig. 3). Implied here is the greater retention of clonidine in the skin of the upper outer thigh than that of either the chest or the upper outer arm.

The total area under the plasma clonidine concentration-time profile (AUC) is a measure of the extent of drug absorption. Figure 4 shows the mean data for the AUC observed following application of the transdermal system to the different skin sites plotted against the mean estimated amount of clonidine released from the system during the 7-day application. The latter values were calculated as the difference between the amount of clonidine in the original system (2.64 mg) and that remaining after the application. The differences in both AUC and amount released were statistically significant between all three sites in the order chest > upper outer arm > upper outer thigh. The high correlation between AUC and amount released indicates that the former reflects quantitatively the latter.

The present study with clonidine supports the previous general observation that the permeability of the skin varies widely between different regions of the body (Feldman et al., 1967). Of the three sites studied, the chest appears the most permeable and the thigh the least permeable, although such differences may *not exist in all sub-*

jects. Differences between the chest and upper outer arm were observed but whether these differences are *clinically significant* remains to be determined.

References

Arndts D, Doevendans J, Kirsten R and Heintz B (1983) New aspects of the Pharmacokinetics and Pharmacodynamics of clonidine in man. Europ J Clinical Pharmacol 24:21–30.
Arndts D, Stahle H and Forster H-J (1981) Development of a RIA for clonidine and its comparison with the reference methods. J Pharmacological Methods 3:103–115.
Feldman RJ and Maibach H-J (1967) Regional variation in percutaneous penetration of ^{14}C-cortisol in man. J Invest Derm 48:181–182.

Correspondence:

Professor M. Rowland
Department of Pharmacy
University of Manchester
Manchester M13 9PL
U.K.

Discussion

SAMBHI:
Did you show a slide on blood pressure side-effects?

HOPKINS:
We did not collect the blood pressure data for analysis but as a safety factor to make sure that the volunteer's blood pressure did not drop too low.

DRAYER:
It appears that plasma clonidine concentrations resulting from patches applied to the thigh, declined slightly even before the patch was removed. Can there be changes in the skin after 3–4 days which slow absorption?

HOPKINS:
There may be a practical answer to this; the thigh is the most difficult site to keep something stuck on to for a week, as the patch may become partly dislodged due to rolling over in the night. Such changes may be a reflection of less effective adhesion to the skin.

ALHENC-GELAS:
Did you see a difference in plasma clonidine levels between individuals?

HOPKINS:
Yes.

Clinical experience with clonidine TTS

F. G. McMahon, R. Michael, A. Jain, J. R. Ryan

In this report, we describe two studies of the safety and efficacy of the new anti-hypertensive treatment, clonidine therapeutic transdermal system (CTTS): a short-term study involving 20 patients who received CTTS alone, and a long-term study of eight patients who received both a thiazide diuretic and CTTS.

Short term study

Methodology

The patient characteristics for the initial study are listed in Table 1. Nineteen of the twenty patients were black and six were male. All patients had diagnoses of essential

Table 1. Patient characteristics

Treatment regimen	Number of patients. race/sex	Age* (years)	Height* (inches)	Weight* (pounds)	Duration of hypertension (years)	Concomitant illness
1 Clonidine TTS system	3 { 2B {1M 1F} 1W {−M}	59.00 ±3.60	67.66 ±5.86	186.60 ±29.16	10.40 ±12.97	IDDM – 1 DJD – 1 Chronic sinusitis – 1
2 Clonidine TTS systems	7B {6F 1M}	59.14 ±6.22	66.57 ±3.77	207.00 ±32.39	12.70 ±9.58	DJD – 6 NIDDM – 1 UTI – 1
3 Clonidine TTS systems	10B {7F 3M}	58.44 ±6.36	63.50 ±3.21	169.00 ±34.41	11.05 ±6.97	DJD – 3 MODM – 1 CAD – 1 Fistula in ano – 1 Hyperuricaemia – 1

Index: NIDDM – Non-insulin dependent diabetes mellitus
DJD – Degenerative joint disease
IDDM – Insulin dependent diabetes mellitus
CAD – Coronary artery disease
MODM – Maturity onset diabetes mellitus
UTI – Urinary tract infection
B – Black
W – White
M – Male
F – Female
* Mean ± S.D.

148

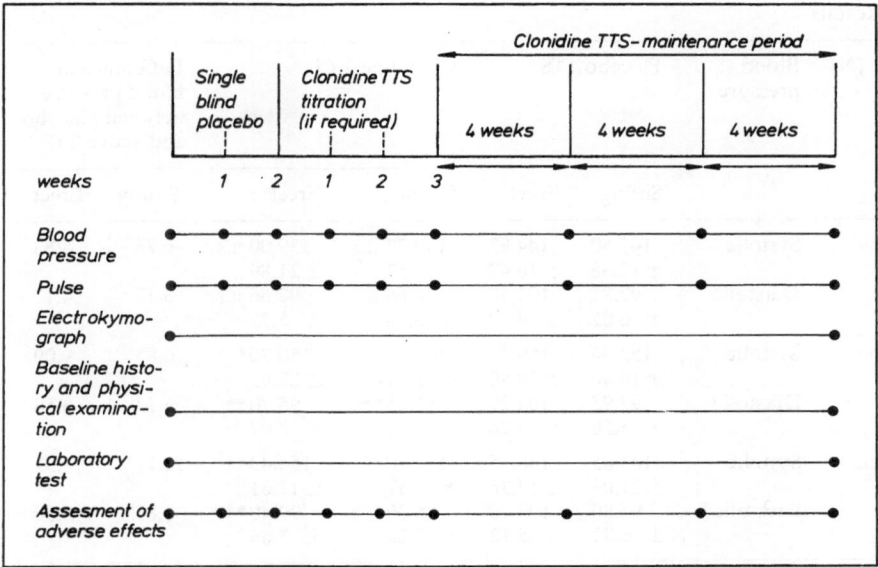

Fig. 1. Protocol for the short-term study.

hypertension; their mean age was 59 years and mean weight approximately 185 pounds. Each CTTS patch contained 2.7 mg of drug and the rate of release was such that 0.1 mg of clonidine was absorbed each 24 hours from each patch.

The design of the first study is shown in Fig. 1. Only patients with mild hypertension (seated diastolic blood pressure of 90–104 mm Hg) were admitted to the study. Patients who had clinically significant concurrent disease or any known allergies were excluded as were women of child-bearing potential. The optimal dose for each subject was found by applying one, two or three CTTS patches during a test period until satisfactory control of blood pressure was achieved. Patches were applied to the upper arm or other hairless area of the torso. Satisfactory control was defined as a reduction in diastolic pressure to less than 90 mm Hg or a 10 mm Hg reduction from baseline values. Optimal doses, once established, were maintained for three months.

Results

The results of the first study are shown in Table 2. It will be noted that three patients responded satisfactorily to a single patch, seven patients required two patches and ten patients required all three patches. Mean blood pressures of patients taking the active drug were reduced by approximately 7/3 mm Hg for the single system in the very mildly hypertensive group, approximately 7/6 mm Hg in those seven patients requiring two systems and approximately 11/7 mm Hg in those teh individuals who required all three patches. Side-effects are shown in Fig. 2. Drowsiness and dry mouth occurred much less frequently with CTTS than would have been expected with oral clonidine. Mild local

Table 2. Results

Treatment (N)	Blood pressure [+]	Placebo TTS		Clonidine TTS		Difference in blood pressure between placebo and active TTS	
		Sitting	Erect	Sitting	Erect	Sitting	Erect
1 Clonidine TTS	Systolic	147.50 ± 17.68	144.83 ± 16.47	140.77 n.s. ± 18.57	139.00 n.s. ± 21.89	6.73	5.83
	Diastolic	97.83 ± 6.82	101.83 ± 4.79	94.66 n.s. ± 6.78	97.66 n.s. ± 5.72	3.17	4.17
(3)							
2 Clonidine TTS	Systolic	152.36 ± 19.40	159.79 ± 19.80	145.50* ± 22.41	150.70* ± 22.93	6.85	9.09
	Diastolic	93.93 ± 3.58	104.29 ± 5.76	87.75** ± 5.72	95.70** ± 8.67	6.17	8.58
(7)							
3 Clonidine TTS	Systolic	163.85 ± 21.06	168.35 ± 17.36	152.70*** ± 21.67	154.43*** ± 17.61	11.15	13.92
	Diastolic	94.80 ± 5.82	104.90 ± 5.12	88.00*** ± 7.28	99.40*** ± 7.64	6.80	5.50
(10)							

[+] Mean ± S.D   n.s. Not significant
*** P 0.005
** P 0.05
* P 0.01

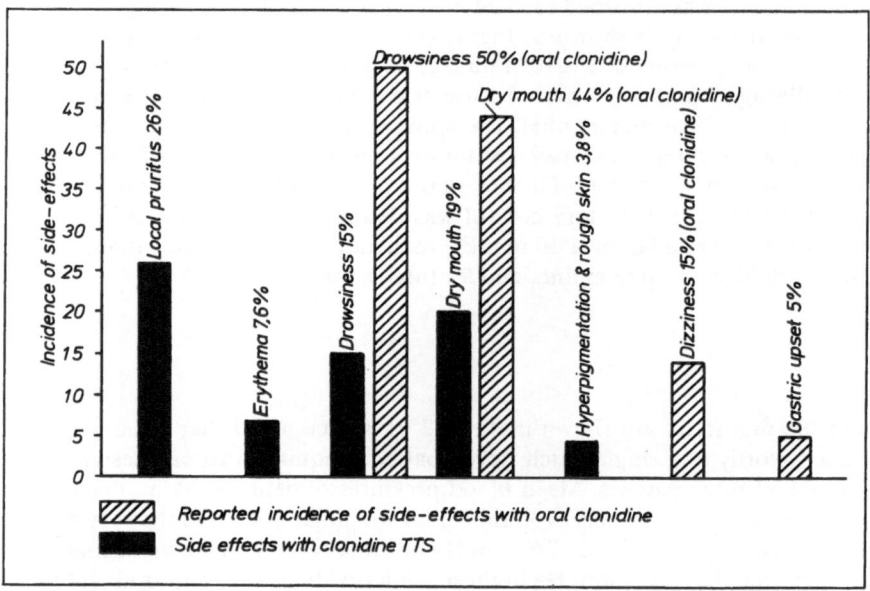

Fig. 2. Incidence of side-effects of CTTS compared with expected incidence of side-effects with oral clonidine.

pruritus occurred in 26% of the study patients but only in one patient did the erythema and pruritis require discontinuation of therapy. We conclude that CTTS given for a period of three months is effective in reducing blood pressure in patients with mild hypertension. This control was achieved even though all but one of our patients were black and therefore the study population was predominantly made up of low renin essential hypertension patients with expanded blood-volume.

Long term study

Methodology

Our second study involved eight patients whose blood pressures were sub-optimally controlled by thiazide diuretics. Patients whose diastolic pressure exceeded 90 mm Hg while being treated with thiazides were admitted to the study. The dose of diuretic was maintained at a constant level and one, two or three CTTS patches were applied as required. Interim results are presented for the first 10 months of the 12 month study period. One patient was lost to follow-up after three months. In the other seven patients the mean blood pressure reduction induced by CTTS was 21/14 mm Hg. Four of the seven patients responded to one patch; three required two patches. As in the first study the side-effects were mild. Dry mouth was noted in three patients and pruritus which did not interfere with treatment was noted in two patients. One patient had to be withdrawn from the study because of moderately severe local pruritic and erythematous reaction after two month's treatment.

Conclusions

Although most patients in these studies had expanded blood volumes (low renin essential hypertension), we have demonstrated that CTTS is effective in reducing blood pressure when used as the sole therapy for a period of three months. Furthermore, this new delivery system can be used effectively in addition to diuretic therapy to give a further decrease in blood pressure. Patient acceptance and compliance were excellent in both studies, although two of our 28 patients (7%) had to be withdrawn from the studies because of localized pruritic erythematous reactions. Apart from this, the systemic side-effects were milder and less frequent than those observed with oral clonidine.

Correspondence:
Dr. F. G. McMahon
Clinical Research Center
134 LaSalle Street
New Orleans
Louisiana 70112
U.S.A.

151

Discussion

SAMBHI:
How good is your evidence that black patients have expanded blood volume?

McMAHON:
Seventy percent of black males in the multicentre study of propranolol and thiazide in hypertension had a low renin level. Also, of the 800 black hypertensives attending our clinic, 40–50% have low renin hypertension.

SAMBHI:
How do you make the jump from there to expansion of plasma volume?

McMAHON:
We think the relationship is well documented in the literature.

PEART:
This is part of the mythology which is owed to John Laragh and it is not true. There is only one consistent finding about blood volume in essential hypertension, and that is that regardless of ethnic origin, there is a reduced plasma volume.

HEILMANN:
The transdermal system provides a balance between the drug input and output which creates an increase in safety for the patient. If you remove the plaster from the skin does the effective level in the blood fall relatively rapidly to non-effective levels? Could there be problems with increased blood pressure after removal of the patch.

McMAHON:
No, as Dr Shaw showed, the blood drug levels gradually fall over two or three days after removal of the patch. Personally I think that clonidine rebound is a much exaggerated phenomenon, but this method of administration will certainly guard against it.

Clinical effectiveness of the transdermal route of antihypertensive treatment

M. A. Weber, J. I. M. Drayer, J. L. Lipson, D. D. Brewer

Introduction

Although it is widely accepted that the treatment of severe hypertension reduces cardiovascular complications, it has only been appreciated recently that treating milder forms of hypertension may also reduce the risk of major cardiac events (Hypertension Detection and Followup Program 1979). There has been some concern that the use of certain drug treatment regimens might lead to a sub-optimal outcome (MRFIT Research Group 1982). Specifically, diuretic agents given to reduce blood pressure might also introduce metabolic risk factors and thereby produce disappointing results (Dollery, 1981). There has been recent interest in non-diuretic single-agent therapy as this approach is simple and potentially safer than diuretic-based therapy. A number of antihypertensive drugs, including beta-blockers and centrally-acting agents, have been shown to be effective in this context (Campese et al. 1980; Drayer et al. 1976; Walker et al. 1982).

The availability of a transdermal system for administering the antihypertensive agent, clonidine, has provided a further method for the treatment of patients with mild to moderate hypertension. This transdermal system, which is described in detail elsewhere in this volume, administers clonidine continuously for a full one-week period. The standard size of patch (3.5 cm²) provides a clonidine dose equivalent to an oral dose of 0.1 mg daily. Plasma clonidine concentrations increase during the first 2 or 3 days of transdermal administration to levels approximately equivalent to mean values seen during oral clonidine treatment (Shaw, in preparation). Thereafter, the concentration appears to remain constant, avoiding the sharp peaks that follow oral administration, and the troughs that occur just before a further oral dose is taken. Thus, it might be anticipated that the systemic side-effects associated with peak plasma drug levels, and the possible loss of blood pressure control associated with the trough levels, would not occur.

In the study described in this report we have evaluated transdermally administered clonidine in 20 patients with mild, uncomplicated, essential hypertension. Our preliminary experience, also reported elsewhere (Weber et al. 1984), has suggested that this method of antihypertensive therapy is effective in this type of patient and appears to be well tolerated.

Methods

The twenty patients participating in the study had essential hypertension. Those with secondary hypertension were excluded by standard clinical and laboratory techniques. The patients were all men, aged 26–68 years (mean 57 years). They had untreated diastolic blood pressures (measured in the supine posture) within the range 91–105 mm Hg. Patients with known heart disease, airway disease, renal or hepatic disease, or endocrine conditions such as diabetes were excluded. Each patient signed an informed consent form in accordance with the Institutional Review Board of the Veterans Administration Medical Center, Long Beach. During the study, the patients were treated with clonidine or placebo, impregnated into self-adhesive skin patches, 3.5 cm² in diameter. These delivery systems were positioned on the skin at weekly intervals throughout the study. The patients could use any part of their upper body (above the umbilicus), but usually chose the anterior chest wall or shoulder. The study began with a 2-week placebo period during which the delivery systems contained no active drug. It was necessary for the blood pressure measured at the end of this phase to be within the range 91–105 mm Hg for the patients to remain in the study. During the first week of the active treatment period, the patients wore one skin patch. If the seated diastolic blood pressure was reduced to less than 90 mm Hg or by at least 10 mm Hg. the patient continued to receive treatment at this dose for a further 3 months. If the blood pressure did not satisfy these criteria after one week, the patient wore two patches for the second week of this titration period and, if necessary, three patches for the third week. Only those patients whose blood pressures were satisfactorily controlled remained in the study for the full 3 month period. The final section of the study was a placebo period during which placebo patches were substituted for the active treatment devices without the knowledge of the patients.

Blood pressure was measured with a standard mercury sphygmomanometer. Blood samples and 24-hour urine collections were obtained at the end of the initial placebo period and at the end of the active treatment period. Routine analysis of plasma biochemistry was performed and plasma renin activity was measured by radio-immunoassay (Sealey et al. 1975). Whole-day aldosterone excretion was measured by immunoassay (Sealey et al. 1972). Statistical comparisons were made by the paired Student's t-test. Values are expressed as mean ± SEM.

Results

Of the 20 patients who entered the study and received active treatment, 12 (60%) achieved the required decrease in seated diastolic pressure.The other eight patients were excluded at the end of the initial titration period and were subsequently treated with conventional antihypertensive agents. One of the 12 remaining patients was being treated with a single therapeutic system, five with two systems, and six with three systems. The mean systolic blood pressure of all 20 patients fell from 138.3±3.3 mm Hg to 134±2.7 mm Hg. The mean diastolic blood pressure fell from 96.9±0.9 mm Hg to 90.8±1.2 mm Hg ($p < 0.001$). Neither heart rate nor body weight changed with treatment. (Mean values before and after treatment were 71±2 bpm and 72±1 bpm, and 81±3 kg and 81±3 kg, respectively). For the 12 patients classified as responders, the mean systolic and diastolic blood pressures at the end of the titration period were 129±3 mm Hg and 87±1 mm Hg respectively. For these 12 patients the mean diastolic blood pressures were 96±3 mm Hg at the end of the pre-treatment placebo period and 98±4 mm Hg at the end of the post-treatment placebo period. There was no significant difference between these two values. The mean of the lowest diastolic blood pressures

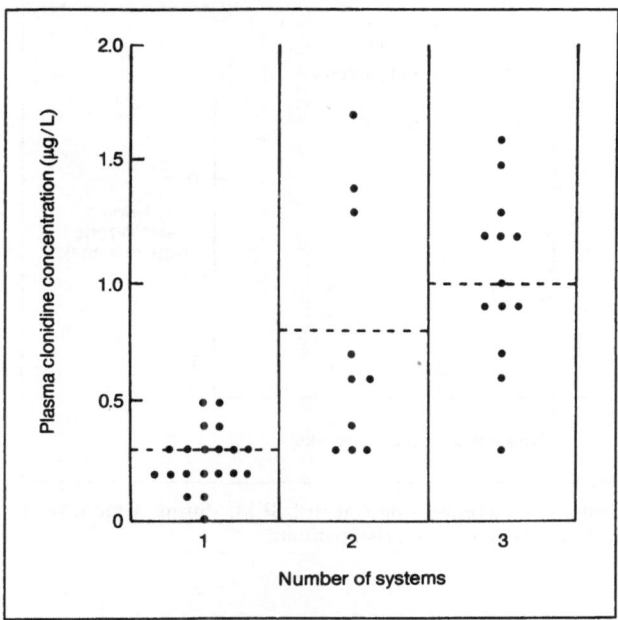

Fig. 1. Plasma concentrations of clonidine during treatment with one, two, or three clonidine transdermal systems.

recorded during the study for each of the twelve patients was 86±2 mm Hg. This value was significantly different from both the pre-treatment and post-treatment placebo values (p < 0.001).

None of the patients in the study discontinued treatment because of adverse effects. Of the 20 patients who received active treatment, six complained of dry mouth (all of a mild degree) and three complained of drowsiness (again of mild degree). Rarely did these side-effects persist for more than one week of treatment. Two of the patients complained of mild pruritis and experienced erythema under their skin patches. In both cases the erythema disappeared within two days of removal of the patch. Plasma clonidine concentrations were measured by radioimmunoassay (Arndts et al. 1982) at different stages of the study. These results are summarized in Fig. 1. The concentrations during the active treatment period were all significantly greater (p < 0.01) than during the placebo periods. The clonidine levels of patients using two or three patches were each significantly greater than those using on patch (p < 0.02 in each case), but were not significantly different from each other. Measurements of plasma renin activity and of urinary aldosterone excretion during the study are shown in Fig. 2. Both of these values decreased significantly during the course of the study. Table 1 shows the routine biochemical measurements taken during the study for the 12 patients completing the protocol. There were no significant changes in plasma concentrations of creatinine, urea nitrogen, sodium or potassium. There was a small but significant decrease in serum uric acid. The 24-hour urinary sodium excretion did not change, indicating that dietary sodium intake remained relatively constant throughout the study.

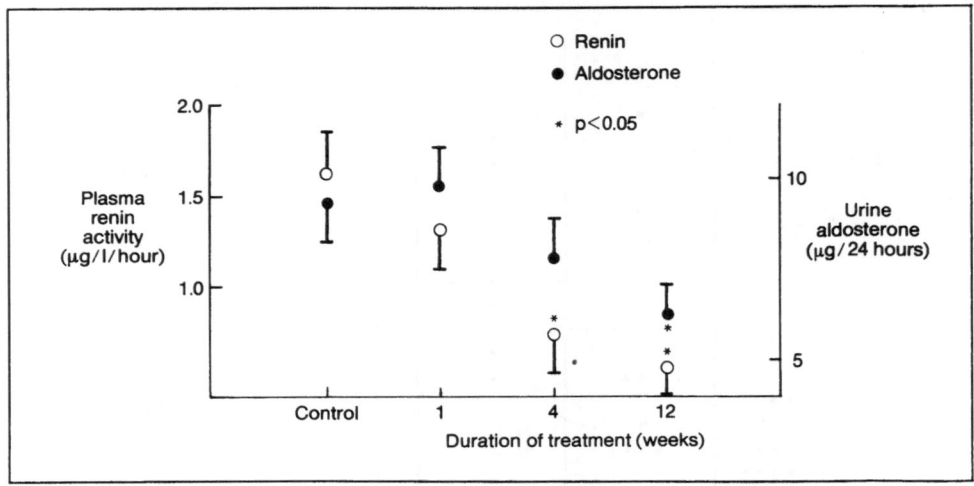

Fig. 2. Plasma renin activity and aldosterone excretion rate (mean ± SEM) during 3 months of treatment with clonidine transdermal systems in 12 hypertensive patients.

Table 1. Laboratory values during treatment with transdermal clonidine

		Placebo	1 month	3 months
Serum urea nitrogen	(mg/l)	158± 9.0	158± 9.0	162±10.0
Serum creatinine	(mg/l)	12± 0.4	13± 0.5	11± 0.4
Serum uric acid	(mg/l)	63± 3.0	60± 4.0	53± 3.0*
Serum sodium	(meq/l)	141± 6.0	140± 0.9	141± 0.8
Serum potassium	(meq/l)	4.5 ± 1.0	4.6 ± 1.0	4.6 ± 1.0
Urinary sodium	(meq/24 hours)	117±14	145±21	119±13

Values are mean ± SEM, n = 12
* p < 0.01

Discussion

In this study we have found that transdermally administered clonidine can normalize blood pressure (i.e. decrease diastolic blood pressure to less than 90 mm Hg) in approximately 60% of patients with mild essential hypertension. When the active treatment was replaced by placebo there was a significant increase in the blood pressure to levels that were not significantly different from the pre-treatment control levels. The side-effects of treatment were generally of short duration and appeared to be milder than those reported previously with oral antihypertensive agents of this type (Schultz et al. 1981).

The plasma clonidine concentrations achieved with the transdermal system were similar to those reported previously with oral clonidine (Arndts et al. 1982). However, as reported by Shaw (in preparation), plasma clonidine concentrations can be sharply elevated shortly after oral administration. It is unlikely that such changes occur during treatment with the transdermal system, and it is thus not surprising that our patients were without noteworthy systemic side-effects during treatment. Clonidine is known to have inhibitory effects on renin release and on the excretion of aldosterone (Weber et al. 1976). The significant reduction in plasma renin activity and aldosterone excretion rates measured in the present study are consistent with the earlier findings, and support the hypothesis that transdermally administered clonidine produces the same clinical and endocrine effects that have been observed in earlier studies with the oral form. During this short-term study no abnormalities were detected by routine biochemical analysis.

The data in this report are very similar to those obtanied during a recent multi-centre study of a large number of patients (Weber et al. in press). The largerscale study also found that diastolic blood pressure could be controlled by transdermal clonidine in at least 60% of patients with mild essential hypertension. The proportion of patients classified as responders, and the absolute decreases in blood pressure were similar in the two studies. Boekhorst (1983) switched oral clonidine treatment to the transdermally administered form in a group of hypertensive patients. There was no loss of blood pressure control despite a tendency for plasma clonidine concentrations to be somewhat lower during the transdermal phase than during the oral treatment. There was a clear decrease in the severity of symptomatic side-effects once the transition in therapy had been accomplished. There has not yet been sufficient long-term experience with transdermally administered clonidine to draw firm conclusions concerning its clinical value, but these early studies suggest that it is an effective and well-tolerated form of treatment. It is possible that these characteristics will help enhance patient compliance with treatment, and that this new method for delivering antihypertensive therapy might become useful in the long-term treatment of patients with mild to moderate essential hypertension.

Summary

The recent development of a transdermal system capable of providing a full week of treatment with clonidine in a single administration has provided a new approach to treating patients with mild to moderate hypertension. We have used the transdermal clonidine system in 20 hypertensive patients for periods of up to 3 months. Twelve patients responded with a decrease in diastolic blood pressure to less than 90 mm Hg. Moreover, the blood pressures during the treatment period were significantly lower than those during either pre- or post-treatment placebo periods. Side-effects of this form of treatment appeared to be milder than during conventional oral treatment. The transdermal method of antihypertensive drug administration appears to be effective and well tolerated, and might be of value in the clinical management of hypertensive patients.

References

1 Arndts D, Stahle H, Forster HJ (1982) Development of a RIA for clonidine and its comparison with the reference methods. J Pharmacol Methods 6:295–307.
2 Boekhorst JC (data on file, Boehringer Ingelheim Ltd.).

3 Campese VM, Romoff M, Telfer N, Weidmann P, Massry SG (1980) Role of sympathetic nerve inhibition and body sodium-volume state in the antihypertensive action of clonidine in essential hypertension. Kidney Int 18:351–357.
4 Dollery CT (1981) Does it matter how blood pressure is reduced? Clin Sci 61:413s–420s.
5 Drayer JIM, Keim HJ, Weber MA, Case DB, Laragh JH (1976) Unexpected pressor responses to propranolol in essential hypertension. Am J Med 60:897–903.
6 Hypertension Detection and Follow-Up Program Cooperative Group (1979) Five-year findings of the hypertension detection and follow-up program. JAMA 242:2562–2571.
7 Multiple Risk Factor Intervention Trial Research Group. Multiple risk factor intervention trial. JAMA 248:1465–1477.
8 Schultz HS, Chretien SD, Brewer DD, Weber MA (1981) Centrally-acting agents in the treatment of hypertension. In: Weber MA (ed.) Treatment Strategies in Hypertension. Symposia Specialists, Miami 191–227.
9 Sealey JE, Buhler FR, Laragh JH, Manning EH, Brunner HR (1972) Aldosterone excretion: physiological variations in man measured by radioimmunoassay or double-isotope dilution. Circ Res 31:367–378.
10 Sealey JE, Laragh JH (1975) Radioimmunoassay of plasma renin activity. Semin Nucl Med 5:189–202.
11 Walker BR, Hare LF, Deitch MW, Gold JA (1982) Comparative effects of guanabenz alone and in combination with hydrochlorothiazide as initial antihypertensive therapy. Curr Ther Res 31:764–775.
12 Weber MA, Case DB, Baer L, Sealey JE, Drayer JIM, Lopez-Ovejero JA, Laragh JH (1976) Renin and aldosterone suppression in the antihypertensive action of clonidine. Am J Cardiol 38:825–830.
13 Weber MA, Drayer JIM, McMahon FG, Hamburger R, Shah A, Kirk L (1984) Transdermal administration of clonidine for the treatment of high blood pressure. Arch Int Med (in press).
14 Weber MA, Drayer JIM, Brewer DD, Lipson JL (1984) Transdermal continuous antihypertensive therapy. Lancet (in press).

Correspondence:
Michael A. Weber, M.D.
Hypertension Center W130
VA Medical Center
5901 East Seventh Street
Long Beach, CA 90822 USA
213/498-6892

Discussion

HAYDUK:
You showed a drop in renin levels in your patients, was there a concurrent increase in weight?

WEBER:
No, there was no weight change in our patients and thus no evidence of fluid retention.

Roundtable discussion on the use of transdermal medication: clinical characteristics and skin reactions

SAMBHI:

The papers in this symposium have provided interesting data on the pharmacokinetics of transdermally administered clonidine and have shown its clinical effectiveness in patients with mild to moderate hypertension. I think we should consider whether this form of treatment causes a skin reaction, how often this occurs, how it can be prevented, and what future research should be contemplated.

WEBER:

The main problem in the discussion of skin reactions from a clinician's point of view is one of definition. Mild pruritus or erythema may occur simply because of skin occlusion for a 7 day period. This sort of reaction is perhaps best termed 'irritation', and may not require a more specific description. However, we have also seen more severe forms of reaction that presumably have a true immunological basis. It is not always easy to distinguish between irritation and the more severe reaction, especially as irritation may be a prelude to sensitization. In the multi-centre study we reported earlier in the symposium, about 30% of patients reported some degree of skin reaction on at least one occasion during the study but only about 6% had more severe reactions that required discontinuation of therapy. All these reactions disappeared completely once treatment was stopped, and as far as we know there have been no irreversible changes. Clearly this raises questions of practical clinical importance. If a patient experiences a minor skin reaction, can the transdermal device be safely applied to another part of the body without eliciting a similar or worse reaction? Would it help to change patches more frequently in susceptible patients, perhaps every 3–5 days? If a patient develops an apparent sensitization to transdermal clonidine, could this cause problems with subsequent oral treatment?

SAMBHI:

Is skin pigmentation a factor in the incidence of irritation?

McMAHON:

We have found no evidence that black patients are any more or less susceptible to skin reactions than white patients.

KAPLAN:

I have had an opportunity to study more closely some of the skin reactions of the patients in the multi-centre study mentioned by Dr Weber. Three patients developed moderate erythema. Once developed, the erythema persisted and was evident every time a new patch was administered. Thus, I believe that once a patient is sensitized to transdermal clonidine, this problem will continue as long as transdermal therapy is maintained. These patients were subsequently patch-tested with transdermal systems containing either clonidine or placebo. The patients had erythematous reactions when given the clonidine-containing patches, but not with the placebo patches. I should like to stress that in these patients we are probably looking at something different from the common irritant reaction, which we believe does not recur with a weekly change of patches. The irritant reactions tend to resolve within hours and almost invariably disappear within one day. I believe that the more persistent erythematous reactions are an early clue that a patient may be developing a true sensitization.

HOPKINS:

Has there been any direct skin testing with clonidine?

KAPLAN:

There have been some preliminary tests with clonidine and with the petrolatum that is combined with clonidine in the transdermal patches. Some patients reacted to the clonidine and others to the petrolatum. However, these data are not conclusive. It is possible that it is not clonidine alone that causes the sensitization, but a combination of clonidine and some other constituent of the skin patch, or even the combination of clonidine with one of its own metabolites. These possibilities are now under investigation.

SHAW:

As part of our preliminary studies with the transdermal preparation we carried out a thorough investigation designed to assess the predictability of this system to elicit irritation and sensitization. The studies were performed in normal volunteers repeatedly using the same skin site for 21 days. After two weeks' rest, we rechallenged the same areas. In no instance did we find evidence for irritation or sensitization. Unfortunately, this classical approach to dermatological reactions does not seem to have predicted what actually occurred in clinical practice. We have now observed with the clonidine transdermal system that the problem may begin at any time between six and twelve weeks after treatment is started. I do not believe that clonidine itself is responsible. A long experience with clonidine, orally or intramuscularly, has shown very little allergic reaction. Another method of assessing the allergic potential of a drug is to determine whether workers involved in its manufacture are prone to such problems. There has been very little report of this. I believe we are seeing either the effect of a 'contaminant' in the system, or, as Dr Kaplan has suggested, an interaction between clonidine and some other substance, as yet unidentified.

It should be remembered that during seven days of occlusion, bacteria proliferate on the skin under the patch. It is possible that there is some kind of interaction between these bacteria and clonidine. The inclusion of a bacteriostatic agent in the transdermal system might retard bacterial growth and prevent this action, but this theory has not yet been tested. Another possibility is to change the patch at more frequent intervals, perhpas every 3–5 days. The bacteria do tend to proliferate after the fourth day, and by making the changes more frequently we might be able to circumvent the problem.

HEILMANN:

Perhaps I could just add a comment to what Dr. Shaw has said? For the past 15 years clonidine has been used extensively in Germany in the form of eye drops for the treatment of glaucoma. During this time, allergic reactions have not been seen in association with this treatment, and such features as conjunctivitis, itching of the eyelids, etc., have been notably absent. This observation, though not in itself a proof, is interesting, particularly since these tissues are rather sensitive. It may perhaps provide a pointer towards identification of the problem.

McMAHON:

I think we should get this discussion on the frequency of skin reactions into perspective. Frankly, I am not disappointed with the results we have seen. I think it is a major therapeutic step to be able to simplify medication and make it convenient. Clearly, this adds to treatment compliance and contributes towards the achievement of therapeutic goals. Even if 10–15% of patients cannot be treated in this fashion, a large majority of individuals remains to benefit from this therapeutic approach.

PEART:

I should like to get a picture of the overall side-effect problem. Skin reactions to transdermal clonidine, although apparently mild in most instances, do represent an additional side-effect. One of the main incentives for utilizing this form of treatment is that side-effects associated with oral treatment, problems such as dry mouth or drowsiness, might be reduced. My concern is whether the benefits we achieve by decreasing these side-effects justify the possible skin problems produced by the transdermal treatment.

WEBER:

Our multi-centre study did not involve sufficient patients, nor a long enough treatment period, to make definitive statements about the frequency of adverse effects. However, no patients dropped out of the study because of dry mouth, drowsiness, or any of the other side-effects seen with most antihypertensive agents. It should be remembered that with just about any antihypertensive agent that has previously been investigated 8–10% of patients are forced to discontinue therapy. Therefore, I believe that the transdermal treatment has brought about a clear benefit. Obviously, it is wise not to persist with this form of treatment in patients who experience symptomatic or worrying skin reactions, but for those who can comfortably tolerate this form of therapy there is a demonstrable advantage in the convenience which it provides.

PEART:

It is characteristic of sensitization that changes in the immunological system can take a long time to develop. Therefore it is possible that a progressively higher percentage of patients might exhibit sensitization as treatment continued. This is not inevitable, but I should like to know whether there is any evidence that the clonidine transdermal system might cause sensitization at a late stage of treatment.

McMAHON:

We have been treating several patients for at least ten months. Some of them did develop erythema or pruritis, but I am not certain whether these changes have been developing as a function of time. As we discussed earlier, I have noted that if these reactions occur, they tend to do so about 4–5 days following administration of the skin patch. In most of these cases, however, I wasn't certain whether we were dealing with a true immunological process or a non-specific inflammatory response.

KAPLAN:

Our experience has been that most patients with unequivocal skin reactions have been diagnosed as having contact dermatitis on skin biopsy studies. We believe that most sensitive patients will be discovered within the first few months of treatment. The remaining resistant patients will be able to continue with therapy for indefinite periods with only a low risk of developing this problem. The data we have compiled so far in the United States seems to support that idea. Of 15 patients who have had at least a year of treatment with transdermal clonidine, only one has developed a late stage dermatological problem.

DE CASPARIS:

Studies in The Netherlands appear to support this. Of 20 patients studied with transdermal clonidine, three were forced to drop out of the study at between 3 and 7 months of treatment because of suspected allergic reactions. The other 17 patients have been treated for up to 15 months, and there has been no further case of an allergic reaction.

SAMBHI:

What is the possibility of desensitizing some of these patients?

SHAW:

Before we can consider such an approach, we must identify the factor causing the sensitization problems. At present, our approach is to try and prevent the problem. If we are able to discover the factor that is producing the sensitization, or perhaps interacting with clonidine to cause the problem, we would hope to eliminate it from the preparation.

TUCK:

There are some patients who seem very satisfied with oral medication. Have people who have participated in studies with transdermal clonidine been asked whether they preferred the oral or transdermal methods?

WEBER:

Some patients definitely preferred using the skin patch, but our overall impression was that most patients didn't have a strong preference either way. I believe that most individuals who are told that they have hypertension, and that they will require lifelong treatment, will soon become adjusted to the problem and will not see taking tablets as a major inconvenience. I feel that the greatest advantage of the transdermal system is not the convenience of once-weekly administration, but the minimization of symptomatic side-effects. In our study there was a small group of patients who had previously been given oral antihypertensive agents that had produced unacceptable side-effects, and for whom the transdermal preparation represented the only acceptable way in which they could be treated with a centrally-acting antihypertensive agent. I am certain that some patients will be most happy to use the transdermal preparation once it becomes available, but I am also certain that many patients now taking oral clonidine will wish to remain with that form of treatment.

MANCIA:

Most people appear to assume that treatment compliance would improve with transdermal clonidine. Is there any hard evidence for this?

McMAHON:

We have always assumed that compliance will be improved by simplying a treatment regimen. This has been true of oral medication taken on a twice-daily basis rather than on a three or four times daily basis. I am optimistic that once-a-week therapy is going to be even easier to comply with than anything we have available at present, but I agree that careful objective studies should be performed to examine this question.

MANCIA:

I wonder whether a week between administering skin patches might be rather long, and whether there might be a danger that patients could forget to change the old patch for a new one. If the patch is left on for too long, or if there is an interval between treatments, will there be a loss in blood pressure control.

DE CASPARIS:

We have some data to suggest that if the patch is left on longer than a week, the plasma concentrations of clonidine do not fall immediately. At present we are doing a study to determine what happens to plasma clonidine levels if the patches are left on for 11 days. I should like to emphasize a point made in an earlier paper dealing with pharmacokinetics. There does appear to be a benefit of transdermal therapy in that there is a constant clonidine level throughout 24 hours, whereas with oral therapy clonidine level is continually changing. We believe that preliminary data indicate that blood pressure control during transdermal therapy is as good as during oral therapy despite an apparently lower mean blood concentration of clonidine.

SAMBHI:

This is an important point, for it suggests that there is no loss of therapeutic efficacy with the constant but generally lower clonidine blood levels achieved with transdermal administration, but there does appear to be a reduction in the incidence of side-effects. I think we can summarize by saying that we believe that this new mode of therapy has some encouraging possibilities, and we are awaiting with interest the data from current investigations to give us further information of the long-term safety and efficacy of the transdermal administration of clonidine.

Panel-Discussion: the role of clonidine in the treatment of mild hypertension

SAMBHI:

I want to make two short comments. Clonidine was introduced in 1966. A year later a paper was published entitled 'The use of clonidine in mild hypertension' which provided statistics about the number of people who responded successfully and the number who did not. The range of blood pressures in those patients extended up to 230/120 mm Hg. In 1967, people must have been quite liberal in their definition of mild hypertension. The second point is that, like many other drugs, when clonidine was first introduced it was used in atrociously high dosages and I think some of the serious side-effects which occurred were the result of those high dosages. Personally I think that a lot of relearning needs to be done about this drug, including a fresh look at it as a candidate for initial therapy in mild hypertension.

I am going to start by asking Dr Mathias if he can provide the experience from St Mary's or from the entire UK if that is what he chooses to do.

MATHIAS, UK:

If we are considering mild hypertension we begin with a choice. Do we treat or do we not treat? This question will be answered more completely be the current MRC trial. Assuming that we decide to treat we have a choice of at least four types of agent which may be used either as monotherapy or combination therapy. I will concentrate upon monotherapy. The desirability of the use of diuretics and beta-blockers we have covered in depth already. The calcium antagonists may be successfully used but side-effects such as tachycardia, flushing and constipation must be taken into consideration. When considering clonidine as monotherapy for mild hypertension we must, as with all drugs, be aware of the balance between side-effects and benefits. This appears to have been favourably affected by the introduction of the TTS system. There certainly are patients to whom the multiple and diverse therapeutic effects of clonidine might be of value. For example the mild hypertensive with migraine or flushing might find that clonidine would help both problems.

McMAHON, New Oreleans:

Fifty percent of mild hypertensives on drugs in the USA are on combination drugs. It is not surprising that patients given any drug as a monotherapy, require a second drug after a period of a month or so. Not so long ago we published a report on the use of a combination drug which has a small dose of clonidine, with a small dose of chlorthalidone. As we have seen earlier the incidence of side-effects is correlated with the rapid changes in the blood drug levels. When the drug was given at bedtime people did not wake up with a dry mouth, neither did they complain of feeling drowsy. I think we need a whole spectrum of drugs. Certainly thiazides are not suitable for everybody and neither are beta-blockers. Hypertension is primarily a disease of the elderly and I worry a great deal about giving beta-blockers to the elderly because of diminished psychic, pulmonary and cardiac function, peripheral vascular disease and so on. I find clonidine an excellent drug to use in the elderly hypertensive patient – as monotherapy or with a thiazide diuretic. The role of calcium antagonists has yet to be defined. The same situation is true of converting enzyme inhibitors. I believe that there is a legitimate role for double combinations as initial therapy. The Food and Drug Administration does not agree with that – they require that you begin titrating with one drug and only then add others. I believe that this is a primitive and obsolete system. Fifty percent of physicians use fixed combinations, although others may disagree with this procedure.

MANCIA, Italy:

I fully agree with what was said yesterday about the need for more individualized treatment. I agree that we should not limit ourselves to diuretics and beta-blockers which have their own serious problems. The MRC trial will probably support this when the results are published. Clonidine has its role as a first drug treatment and in fact in Italy we use it in this manner. We do not use a combination. We use slow release clonidine once a day and we find it quite satisfactory in the treatment of moderate and mild hypertension. We have shown that the blood pressure is reduced throughout the full 24-hour period. There is a similar reduction in heart rate so the double product is also reduced. We have very few problems with side-effects when we use slow release clonidine once a day. It is not the only drug we use, of course, but it is one of the drugs we use as a first-step approach.

SAMBHI:
Dr Hayduk, may we have your comments and in addition to giving me your opinion please tell us why clonidine has been so unpopular in Germany?

HAYDUK, German:
I am sure that clonidine was only unpopular because it was given in doses as high as 300 µg six times daily. Patients receiving these quantities certainly were drowsy and complained of dry mouth. At the time we, in Germany, thought that the escape phenomenon was important here but you never see this with low dose clonidine. We would not have considered high dose clonidine as a first-step treatment of mild hypertension but in a low dose it does not have worse metabolic effects than beta-blockers or thiazides. Now I would give clonidine, as the normal drug, in a slow release form or in TTS, even in mild hypertension. I would also give clonidine with a thiazide in a fixed combination, because the patient does not count the substances he is prescribed, he only counts the pills.

GUTHRIE, U.S.A.
We have been especially concerned about the latent metabolic risks of long-term pharmacotherapy. This is not so important in older patients, but younger patients may be exposed to these drugs for many years. Clonidine does not appear to carry many potential risks, and for that reason we have been attracted to it as first drug therapy. Another very special subgroup of patients with mild hypertension is those with diabetes mellitus. There is no evidence that clonidine adversely affects glucose tolerance, therefore we have been attracted to its use in the treatment of these patients.

FRANKLIN, U.S.A.:
The first session showed that central alpha$_2$-agonists appear to work on the sympathetic nervous system, attaining good blood pressure control without sacrificing baroreceptor control and without gross abnormalities in haemodynamic function. It is possible that a more optimal metabolic profile is obtained than with other agents. This is certainly very attractive for hypertensive therapy. The major drawbacks appear to be sedation and dry mouth. It seems that tailoring the approach to suit the individual is extremely important for patient acceptance. I think this requires smaller doses, perhaps the use of a single dose in the elderly, where metabolic changes result in a longer half-life. A combination of smaller doses of clonidine with a diuretic could also be used when necessary and, of course, TTS will be useful when it is available. This will give us a variety of different approaches, which we can use to get over this large stumbling block of sedation and dry mouth. I think that in the next few years studies on hypertension will be focusing on the potential side-effects and risks of diuretics and other agents. New investigations will be designed to compare one agent against another and I think they will provide very important guidelines for future choice of antihypertensive agents.

HAYDUK:
I think what we have learned from clonidine is that when it is used in very low doses it is extremely effective. Drugs such as alpha methyl dopa and clonidine lower the heart rate a little and although they may not provide cardiac protection like the beta-blockers it is likely that they may cause similar effects. Some cardiologists even claim that these drugs may be better than beta-blockers in this respect. Unlike diuretics and beta-blockers clonidine does not interfere with carbohydrate metabolism and probably does not interfere with lipid metabolism. There are quite a few reasons for using clonidine as a first-line drug and to consider it safe from all these points of view. Echocardiographic studies have shown that drugs which stimulate the sympathetic nervous system, such as diuretics and vasodilators, are not likely to help patients who have hypertension and left ventricular hypertrophy. Their blood pressure might come down but there will not necessarily be a regression of their hypertrophy. On the other hand, drugs which modulate the sympathetic

nervous system such as alpha methyl dopa and clonidine, may both lower blood pressure and cause regression of hypertrophy. The action of beta-blockers in this situation is not yet clarified. This may be yet another reason or the inclusion of sympatholytic agents in antihypertensive treatment, even if only in a low dose. With clonidine we know that we can achieve blood pressure control with a low dose.

SAMBHI:
That's a very good point. To which studies were you referring?

HAYDUK:
There are a number of studies. We have done quite a few studies with echocardiography and left ventricular hypertrophy; we have used diuretics, vasodilators and some beta-blockers; we are now working on alpha methyl dopa, clonidine and converting enzyme inhibitors.

WEBER U.S.A.:
I do not have much to add about clonidine but I do want to make one quick comment which I think ought to be made in a symposium which purports to be talking about mild hypertension. It goes back to some of the data that Professor Peart showed in his introductory talk. We know that when children pass through puberty, their blood pressure tends to be in the region of 90/ 60 mm Hg. Probably increases from that level are not inevitable and might be reflections of all sorts of events. It is not surprising, therefore, that the slide which Prof. Peart showed yesterday morning, based on life insurance actuarial data, indicates a continuum of risk. The lower one's blood pressure, the better off one is. A blood pressure of 120/80 mm Hg which approximates to the standard risk is fine, but if your pressure is only 90/60 mm Hg you are a lot better off. If I remember correctly, those with a blood pressure of 90/60 mm Hg have about 70% of the risk of those with 120/80 mm Hg. So to my simple way of looking at things, I think that those with a blood pressure of 120/80 mm Hg might be described as already having mild hypertension and at the level of 140/100 mm Hg, that we are cheerfully talking about as being mild hypertension, the problem might already be quite serious. I wonder if one of the reasons that these studies of so-called mild hypertension have not seemed all that effective is because all they have been doing is taking people with unsatisfactory blood pressure and making it just slightly less unsatisfactory. Perhaps they have not been getting near to what the goal of the blood pressure reduction should be. What I hope to gain from further discussions of mild hypertension are methods of bringing blood pressure down to some sort of optimal level. I think there is a great deal more to be done in the treatment of hypertension in more aggressive and creative ways.

SAMBHI:
I would like to make two points. Number one, when you elect a Commander General, he sets the pace. It was Professor Peart who decided not to talk about mild hypertension; he set the boundaries to our discussion. Number two, I take your point about the risk but, although it is true that there is greater risk associated with a blood pressure of 120/80 mm Hg than with one of 110/ 70 mm Hg let us not make the mistake of assuming that you can bestow the same benefit by induced reduction of blood pressure. People with a blood pressure of 110/70 mm Hg have it because they have a natural elasticity and compliance of the cardiovascular system, you cannot necessarily bestow that by induced pharmacological reduction of blood pressure. Where you have stenotic lesions it can be dangerous to reduce blood pressure because flow beyond the lesion would be inadequate. Lowering the blood pressure of a 55-year-old man will not make him a 21-year-old.

MANCIA:
We are paying a price for standing up. You need pressure in non-compliant vessels.

WEBER:
We do not know that.

PEART:
If you can persuade somebody to provide you with the 5 million dollars it is going to cost to mount a very small trial of lowering pressure of 130/90 mm Hg to 90/60 mm Hg, I think you will be very lucky.

HAYDUK:

A recent study in elderly hypertensives reduced blood pressure from about 200/100 mm Hg to about 130/80 mm Hg which by your criteria is not even normal. After 3 days, no-one could get out of his bed.

FRANKLIN:

The casual blood pressure level on which the acturial data is dependent is group probability. Whereas this is very satisfactory in setting rates for insurance it is not satisfactory for physicians in the determination of individual risks for their patients.

CEREMUŻIŃSKI, Poland:

I believe that clonidine has some special indications. I would regard clonidine to be the drug of choice when hypertension is associated with angina pectoris, hyperkinetic syndrome, borderline hyperthyroidism, or a high level of anxiety. All these conditions are fairly common in contemporary society.

Concluding remarks

W. S. Peart

The aims of this workshop were to survey the action of the central and peripheral nervous systems in mild hypertension and to review the status of current research in the field. As a result we have all learned a great deal about recent developments in the understanding of the neuropharmacology and physiology of the nervous system. Increased knowledge in this field has led to a resurgence of interest in drugs such as clonidine which act centrally on the nervous system. This area was, therefore, an important focus of attention of the workshop.

It has been customary to treat high blood pressure with a variety of drugs. We thought we understood their modes of action. In many cases, however, it is clear that this is not the case. For example, we have been using thiazides to lower blood pressure for 20 years. These drugs act quickly and effectively but we do not know how they work. As far as clonidine is concerned, one reason for my interest in this drug is because of its striking central effect in circumstances where I would not expect it to work. It brings the influence of the central pathways in the brain into prominence. An extreme example in this area is in the treatment of patients with phaeochromocytoma. I had thought that high blood pressure in phaeochromocytoma was maintained mainly by circulating levels of noradrenaline even though I had been unable to lower blood pressure with alpha-blockade in some of these patients. Now I must conclude that other, secondary, factors had come into play in such patients. As you know, blood pressure does not drop in all patients when the primary cause of the hypertension, whether it be phaeochromocytoma, Conn's syndrome, unilateral renal disease or Cushing's syndrome, is removed. It became conventional to believe that this secondary phenomenon was present in the kidney or blood vessels. For example, pathological changes in the blood vessels might be responsible for the maintenance of high blood pressure. I became very impressed, therefore, by the fact that clonidine lowered the blood pressure in patients with phaeochromocytoma and further impressed by its ability to lower the blood pressure in what I had thought was primarily a humoral effect of the kidney on the circulation. This led me to re-examine my views on the factors which were maintaining the circulation, as revealed by clonidine. There is a need for a great deal more work in this area and the contributions to the workshop indicate that progress is already being made.

A large amount of clinical and experimental data on the use of clonidine was presented at the workshop. It was clear that although clonidine has been available for some time, only now are we learning how to use it with the greatest safety and effect. There is a fashion for the use of every drug and as soon as a new drug is introduced, each physician has to learn from his own experience what are its uses and limitations. In the past, however, there has been a tendency to prescribe drugs only at the dose initially recommended. I feel that physicians have not experimented enough but clinical pharmacologists are also to blame. They have, perhaps, given undue emphasis to drug metabolism and plasma levels and neglected the observation that the action of each drug has a biological component which is not necessarily directly related to the plasma level. For example, if propranolol had been viewed only in that way, it would not have been discovered that the effect of a single dose on heart rate may last for 24 hours in many patients and therefore a long-acting preparation is unnecessary. Now we are returning to low dose clonidine just as we returned to low dose thiazides. In most patients it is 6 weeks before the effect of thiazides reaches maximum, so patience is required. We must learn not to follow fashion but to experiment with drugs.

Clonidine has been on the market for a long time but only now are we investigating it in sufficient detail and learning the importance of low dose clonidine.

A number of presentations concerned a new transdermal method of drug administration. The principle of this has been known for centuries. For instance, the use of goose grease to facilitate the passage of substances through the skin was a familiar practice in folk medicine. Every old sailor who chewed tobacco was aware that he did it for the central effects of the tobacco but drug administration by buccal lozenges is a recent development. Similarly, the effects of taking snuff were known for many years before drugs such as vasopressin were administered nasally. The information has been available for a long time but we have neglected it. This seems to be the history of medicine and indeed of mankind: information is available from daily life that could be beneficial if only we had the wit to make use of it. We have heard some of the difficulties associated with the transdermal application of clonidine but I am not too worried about them because I see them as problems that are there to be solved. I am sure they will be solved and out of it will come better knowledge of clonidine and of therapy in mild hypertension.

Acknowledgements

It is a pleasure to thank all the speakers and Boehringer Ingelheim for an excellent workshop.

Participants

Dr F. Alhenc-Gelas
Hôpital Broussais
Medecine 8
96 rue Didot
75674 Paris
France

Professor L. Ceremużyński
Department of Cardiology
Warsaw Postgraduate School
Grochowski Hospital
04-073 Warsaw
Poland

Dr J. G. Collier
Department of Pharmacology
St George's Hospital Medical School
Blackshaw Road
Tooting
London SW17
U.K.

Dr J. I. M. Drayer
Hypertension Center
Veterans Administration Center
5901 East 7th Street
Long Beach
California 90822
U.S.A.

Professor S. S. Franklin
School of Medicine
University of California
Los Angeles
California 90033
U.S.A.

Dr G. P. Guthrie
Department of Medicine
University of Kentucky
College of Medicine
Lexington
Kentucky 40536
U.S.A.

Professor K. Hayduk
Marien-Hospital, Inn. Abt.
Rochusstraße 2
4000 Düsseldorf 30
F.R.G.

Professor K. Heilmann
Beethovenplatz 2
8000 München 2
F.R.G.

Dr K. Hopkins
Medeval Ltd
Coupland III Building
University of Manchester
Oxford Road
Manchester M13 9PL
U.K.

Professor G. Mancia
Via Rontgen 19
Milan
Italy

Dr C. Mathias
St Mary's Hospital
London W2 1NY
U.K.

Professor F. G. McMahon
Head, Therapeutics Section
Tulane University
School of Medicine
1430 Tulane Avenue
New Orleans
Louisiana 70112
U.S.A.

Professor W. S. Peart
St. Mary's Hospital
London W2 1NY
U.K.

Dr R. J. Polinsky
Laboratory of Clinical Science
National Institute of Mental Health
Bethesda
Maryland 20205
U.S.A.

Professor M. Sambhi
Sepulveda Veteran's
Administration Center
161 11 Plummer Street
Sepulveda
California 91343
U.S.A.

Dr J. E. Shaw
Alza Corporation
950 Page Mill Road
Palo Alto
California 94304
U.S.A.

Dr M. L. Tuck
School of Medicine
University of California
Los Angeles
California 90033
U.S.A.

Professor M. A. Weber
Hypertension Center
Veterans Administration Center
5901 East 7th Street
Long Beach
California 90822
U.S.A.

Subject index

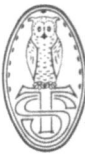